What is a Doctor?

Essays on Medicine and

Human Natural History

What is a Doctor?

Essays on Medicine and

Human Natural History

Alex Comfort, M.B., Ph.D., D.Sc.

George F. Stickley Company
210 West Washington Square
Philadelphia, PA 19106

Manufactured in the United States of America; Published by the George F. Stickley Company, 210 W. Washington Square, Philadelphia, PA. 19106.

Second Printing—February 1981

Some of the essays in this collection have been reprinted from the medical literature: The Journal of Operational Psychiatry, Postgraduate Medicine, Nature, Modern Medicine, and the Western Journal of Medicine.

Contents

Life is short, skill is long—the time for action is fleeting, trial and error is risky, clinical judgment is difficult. Not only must the physician do his office: the patient, the bystanders and the environment must also play their parts.

HIPPOCRATES

Everything in the world and in Man must be implicit in the physician. Herein lies the error of those who do not understand the physician aright.

PARACELSUS

Introduction

That these are "collected essays" neither can nor need, I think, be disguised. They extend over several years, and I have not altered them to disclaim errors of prediction or remove overlaps. Each stands alone.

The title of the first essay ("What is a Doctor?") has been given intentionally to the whole book. Some might well wonder why—psychiatry is medicine, and sexual counseling and the comprehension of odd phenomena such as masochism are fringe medicine; biology is medicine in the preclinical year, but talk about neurology and epistemology is philosophy and better avoided; and political ethology is not medicine at all. I disagree. The motto of my hospital was "Homo sum, nil humani a me alienum puto"—I'm human: all human business is my business. The business of the present medical curriculum is knowledge, knowledge so wide and so congested that the briefest absence from the assembly line leaves one deficient and in need of Continuing Education. This is splendid—who would wish to practice with only the scientific equipment of Heberden, or even Osler, when he can know so much more? But the business of medicine is knowledge *and* insight *and* clinical judgment, so that no physician fresh from board examinations would be disappointed if he could practice as well as Heberden, or Osler, or even Ambroise Paré, despite their lack of grounding in modern science. Nobody can teach judgment, except by example, but the London Hospital motto has the right idea about one of the prerequisites, a necessary though not a sufficient condition, of insight. So if this book is discursive, I make no apology for that either.

Psychiatrists, which basically I am not, are probably more at ease with the idea of humanistic studies as a professional concern. On the other hand, we have to be leery of "humanistic studies," having seen American, and indeed, world psychiatry reduced to a shambles by the self-indulgent speculation of psychiatrists who were not *physicians*. Much of this era of psychiatric fashion may sink without trace in the growth of neuroendocrine studies. Scientific medicine is a good cathartic for this kind of thing, but its occupational hazard, as it is now taught to students, is tunnel vision. If you cure but don't heal, your patients will go to a quack—the threat of "holistic medicine" laced with pyramidology and rolfing is real enough to stress this point in the United States. Experienced patients who are "into" self-realization and suspect doctors of being—out of their own mouths—only tradesmen with marketable techniques, have a point. If one can show that science can itself be insight-giving, and that insight is a good jumping-off point for clinical judgment and social responsibility, much of the case is made for an examination by practicing and by future physicians of some of the areas of "soft" science which I have included in these papers.

I address this book to students, because they are educable—in the full awareness that faced with finals they may not have the time to read it. Some of my colleagues may like to use it also, though there is no tear-out page for continuing credit at the back. It represents personal experience, not instructional bumptiousness, and one of its functions is to incite collegial disagreement. As in writing about sex education, one cannot write about the background areas of medicine and please everybody.

One part of medicine is beyond all cavil precise knowledge, *expertise*. Nobody is going to cavil about this—not you the reader, for you would not want to consult, nor entrust your spouse or mother to, a doctor who manifestly lacked it: not the dean of any medical school, because our educational system is geared to giving and testing skills of this kind, though often of no other kind: not the A.M.A., because in our society the pretensions, the status and the pay of the doctor depend on the fact that, like an airline pilot, he is the responsible expert, making decisions which affect life and limb—and to such we rightly genuflect.

Expertise—which includes specialization, for not all of us are going into family practice or primary care—is the easiest of the requirements of doctorhood to satisfy. In fact, you will not get out of any American medical school or pass between the upper and the nether millstone of licensure without having some of it. If you are any good as a student you will have a great deal of it—simply through living in the late 20th century you will know more, far more, about the scientific basis of disease and medicine than Hunter, or Hippocrates, or Osler, because you can hardly help doing so.

Clinical judgment is harder, because it involves more variables and is more a test of your own personal makeup than the mere prerequisite, acquisition of knowledge. (We rely on examination-testing of knowledge, in fact, partly to make sure that if you have no clinical judgment you will at least have some information to fall back on.) One can know a hell of a lot of science, read every article in every journal, take continuing medical education to the point of stupor, and still lack clinical judgment. We have all met people who are licensed, learned and loved by patients, and who have absolutely none.

What is clinical judgment? When I was a junior pediatrician, we were often confronted on the outpatient service with the child offered for tonsillectomy, circumcision or the like. The teaching was: "If you think that operation is necessary, send them to A, who removes tonsils and foreskins 'routinely.' If you are satisfied it is not necessary and should not be done, send them to B, who will never operate under any circumstances. If you are genuinely in doubt, send them to C, because he has clinical judgment and will act in the best interest of the child."

A, B, and C were all competent surgeons, but A and B were journey-men like the iceman or the cleaner, to whom one says "do this" and he doeth it. C, by contrast was a surgeon and a *doctor* whose opinion was worth having; he alone could correct the errors of our inexperience.

You cannot teach clinical judgment, though it is contagious, but you can encourage it. The way to acquire it is primarily through role-modeling teachers who have it (it is important not to make a mistake here, or the damage can last throughout your working life) and by self-medication: you have to acquire *insight*.

Now insight is a term-of-art from discursive psychiatry. In the most fanatic model, insight meant agreeing with the interpretations of your analyst, especially if he happened to be your training analyst. I do not use it in that sense. "Analysis" in any of the classical models is highly instructive, and now and again one sees a gynecologist or a plastic surgeon whom one would like to submit to it for the good of his soul and his patients. But most of us are not going that road. Few patients, even, now submit their symptoms to classical analysis, and only the devout practice it by the book. In fact, recommendation of prolonged analysis as a religiomedical panacea is evidence in itself of lack of clinical judgment in the face of patients who have had ten years or more of it, acquired much "insight," and still kept the impotence, the asthma, the ill-temper or the biochemical disorder of thinking or mood which led them to undertake it.

But at least it gave us some useful ideas. The most important for the physician is counter-transference. Transference we all know—the pa-tient incorporates us into his fantasies, unloads his problems on us, and we have to be agile to avoid colluding in this process by playing God, to avoid being angry because the patient identifies us with his parents and expresses hostility to us—and still more agile to see what is happening and make therapeutic use of it before handing back the fantasy of its possessor. Counter-transference is far less popular, be-cause it involves the fantasies we project on the patient. One of those is the fantasy involved in becoming or being a doctor. Nobody is supe-rior to those fantasies, and most of us (apart from a few who simply saw medicine as a license to perform wallet biopsies and own a yacht, and who are properly gangsters rather than doctors, pursuing fantasies of a different order) got into medicine because of them. We may have been—and most of us are—aghast at and afraid of death, and react by the pursuit of cure. Curing disease and postponing death are proper aims of doctoring—but if we don't inspect ourselves we may react by fear and hatred of the patient in whom disease cannot be cured or death postponed. If old age threatens us, we may be constitutionally unable to treat older patients. If we had gender problems we may do a lot of mischief to patients who have them. If we had obscure diffi-culties in our early explorations of the human body we may occupy our practice with what are, to the amazed observer, psychotic assaults on the uterus and pelvic organs, the breasts, and other structures in our devoted patients. Or if we have one of the more diffuse forms of unease which human beings so often experience, we may become grandiose, impatient, authoritarian, overanxious, workaholic, weak-kneed with manipulative patients, or simpering toward dominant patients. In other words, we may need to get wise to ourselves and put away childish things. Medicine is for adults, not neotenic children.

Our medical curricula provide little or no opportunity to get this kind of insight. It has to be gotten young, before our professional fantasy is set in concrete. You cannot impart insight to a departmental chairman, or at least not without truly psychiatric exertion. (If you thought that a cheap shot, recall that the first exercise in getting insight into what we are doing is to get rid of the illusion—which is one of the main attractions of medicine—that we are invulnerable and not as other men and women.)

It is, in fact, attitude, not stupidity or ignorance, which is the main barrier to clinical judgment. Good judgment involves doing that which will make the patient feel better, not that which makes us feel better.

If we accept this—and we had better, if we really want to heal rather than treat—we have to be advised that "insight" is not, like immunization, a one-shot charisma. The next hurdle is *wisdom*. That is still more unsettling. It gives us an image of sententiousness which we all now, having some awareness of past medical moralists and philosophers who made themselves ridiculous in hindsight, want to avoid: Sarastro with a false beard, holding forth about Deeper Realities. All that I mean by "wisdom" is a sensitive attention to ordinary, shallow realities, to the components of human experience, and an awareness of the fact that their diversity and multiplicity are patterned. The best way to get it, if we want to be doctors, is not to study philosophy, unless it interests us to read other men's systems, but to cultivate a consuming interest in human natural history; as an ornithologist lives birds, we need to live and study people.

Knowledge doesn't produce wisdom, any more than it produces insight, but if we are interested in humans we will want to know a great many things besides the relations of the second part of the duodenum and the normal range of blood SGOT. If one treats patients using insight one can't help asking, at some point, what exactly we mean by "I"—when I make up my mind to administer oxygen or move my big toe. Some of us will have a bent toward communication (a dangerous word nowadays because it is often self-indulgent). Others will get interested in anthropology, and the posture our society adopts compared with others who see things differently. We may read up on subatomic physics, and realize that not only is the objective world not so objective after all, but that since what we perceive is largely a function of the way our nervous system works, the nature of the phenomenal world falls in our bailiwick. As citizens we shall have politics forced on us, and as economically privileged citizens we shall have to weigh the pro's and con's of professional liberty and responsibility—which are ordinary liberty and responsibility writ large—against the kind of Neanderthal laissez-faire which is as trendy today as Marxism was in the Thirties.

Wisdom consists in moving clinical judgment up, from the special to the general. If we can get judgment, we can generalize it to secure wisdom, which is why medicine is supposed to be a liberal profession. This involves, at a minimum, reading other things besides trade publications dealing with skills. Some doctors and students, if they have the application to get through the essays in this book, will chuck it away, remarking "What the hell has all this to do with the practice of medicine?" or opine that it's all very fine but they have not learned anything about reducing Mr. Appelbaum's inguinal hernia. That was why I selected the title.

The old preparation for "wisdom" as a cherry on the top of medicine, converting it from apothecary-surgeonship to doctoring, was a liberal education. But since nobody gets one now (a liberal arts course on 100 Great Books or epic poetry in translation is not a substitute so much as an immunizing dose), the modern physician has to shift for himself in the gaps of answering multiple-choice questions. He does not have to be terrific with people, either, to be holistic. It is permitted in medicine, if you really can't talk to other humans, to concentrate on slides or cadavera, but even here your personal foibles will find you out. A necrophiliac does not make a good pathologist, any more than sadists make good surgeons. If you have to choose, then, settle for insight. It will make you less of a menace, and wisdom may come later if you are made that way and susceptible to education.

Some people—colleagues and students—will classify a great deal in this book as "psychiatry," which means that some will greet it with enthusiasm as "their bag" and others reject it as not for them. "Psychiatry" itself excites suspicion among some and intemperate addiction in others. This is because, in our society, psychiatry is grossly overloaded. It really represents three distinct projects. The first is the ability to comprehend human behavior and assist people in dealing with experiences common to the species in this day and society with the resources generally available to humans, although these experiences and resources differ greatly from person to person. This exercise is better called counseling. Many older sources of counseling, such as society, religion, and family have collapsed into a quasi-medical context. All doctors are going to practice "psychiatry" as soon as they speak to, treat, or avoid a patient, and they had better know what is known about it. The second exercise consists in helping those whose posture and experience are basically atypical or distorted by biochemical, emotional and bio-emotional processes in their own heads. This discipline is the treatment of mental pathology. It is best left to those whose business it is, but we all need to be clinically aware of it, or we miss depression and impending suicide, or treat delusional symptoms. The third is the application of psychiatric knowledge to ourselves. No man is well treated if the physician is himself irrational, or unaware of his unreason. Since the first and the third of these undertakings enter every clinical interview, even if it be in orthopedics or hematology, we need the skills involved as part of our professional equipment, and if we do not like to call them psychiatric we had better call them "good medical practice."

Another area of concentration is sexuality. Sex as a human pleasure is no more part of medicine than is good cooking. But sexual dysfunction is, just as indigestion and nutrition and alcoholism are. Moreover, in the role of sole surviving counselors we are going to be expected to deal with it. Since it happens to be a major source of personal disturbance for those who enter medicine—as surveys have shown—we had better be comfortable with it, if only in the interest of insight (let alone the avoidance of mischief such as has been done in the past by tirades about the abnormality of normal behavior, or rash and uncalculated counsel to abstain from intercourse after a heart attack). Of the serious trouble seen in psychiatric sexual practice, about half has originated, in my experience, in the personal discomfort of one of the medical advisors whom the patient has seen, and who did not say the right thing.

So too with the physical and social differences between the sexes. Indeed, in writing this book one groped continuously for some neutral designation intermediate between "he" and "she," since "he" is no longer masculine *and* common and one needs to avoid accusations—misplaced, so far as I am concerned—of sexism, without insufferable stylistic contortion over "persons."

Medicine has as bad a record in recognizing human equality as it has in other socially progressive contexts—women were admitted to practice it almost within living memory. They are still too often attended by male physicians and surgeons with a paternalism which is a disguise for active hostility. The conscientious doctor of either sex is meanwhile besieged by waves of biological, endocrine, political, psychiatric or frankly propagandist comment—in the knowledge that however discriminating the doctor may be in sifting this mass, the patients will have read it, too. He or she will meet women deeply conscious of the social injustices done them, women of conventional tastes who are seriously disturbed by changes in expectation which the new climate imposes, women who desire not only orgasm but a particular kind of orgasm because they have been reading orgasmic theology from one or another source; men expressing or repressing deep hostility to women, men who are badly thrown by their encounter with a partner, formerly submissive, who is now sexually or socially assertive; and, of course, thoroughly confused people—often young people suffering from parental confusion and acting-out—of both sexes. I have looked at some of this confused and confusing background in some of the papers which follow, not from the standpoint of feminism-antifeminism, but rather by trying to examine some of our sources of knowledge, from pulp fiction to "sociobiology." We need all the information about human natural history we can get, whatever its place of origin.

Another such area of personal disturbance with dire clinical effects is our neglect of geriatric medicine. Few doctors cannot stand birth, but a great many cannot stand the sight of old age. None of the ground covered in what follows, then, is dragged in unseasonably to the discussion of medicine. I have picked out some of the areas of our lowest performance, and no expertise in doing bypass operations at open-heart surgery can make up for the deficiency. I would hope that the rationale for these essays will appear in the reading of them.

From what I have said you will appreciate why I have not made this a book of specifically clinical papers—you have enough of such professional information already. Be reassured, however, that I am and always have been a clinician, and regard the clinician as the most genuine and paradigmatic physician. I also spent more than twenty years in laboratory research on the nature of aging processes: I have not written about that here because I have done so at length elsewhere, and though it is on the verge of producing clinical applications—especially in immunology—there are probably several turns of the road ahead before it enters office practice. In addressing gerontology I have had more to say about our attitudes as physicians toward the old—which are relevant now—than about research, which will be relevant later. I have touched at some length on the new universe of quantum physics, not because we are going to apply it at the technical level outside radiology, but because medicine and neurology are still unwittingly Newtonian, like most of our practical, middle-order attitudes. This is probably a good thing for our patients, who are "middle-order" organisms, because of the risk that quantum logic and the universe it implies may go to our heads (if we have weak ones). Football coach realism is a reasonably safe approach compared with others which call for nonintuitive views of reality, but our patients are now apt to have read popularizations of nonintuitive world models, and to have less hesitation in applying them to "mind," "reality" and "existence" than we.

Lastly I have written about politics. If I declared an interest by saying "I am a Republican, a Democrat, a Socialist, a John Bircher" I could at least be sure that my prejudices would be correctly identified. In fact I am an anarchist, and that gives rise to problems at once: "anarchist" in some minds means a violent and disruptive radical. People think of the Baader Meinhof Gang, the Weathermen, and Czolgocz, who shot President McKinley. In fact it simply means someone who thinks that centralized power should be reduced to the practical minimum and individual responsibility increased to the practical maximum—not at all a frightening idea to Americans used to talking about free enterprise. One could have refused combat by using some other name, but the ideology is important to doctors as a professional matter, because it is already implicit in our acceptance of the independence of the physician, his responsibility to the patient, and the patient's inalienable rights. A decent doctor practicing excellent medicine is an ideological "anarchist" whether he likes it or not, and regardless of how, or whether, he votes. The doctor is anarchistic not democratic, mind you—for if the majority vote to withhold treatment from Jews or to kill persons over 70, he will tell the majority to go to the devil, as he should. If the majority's alguazils forbid him the use of certain medications which he considers necessary and beneficial, he will ignore or outwit them, as he should. Recognition of exactly what our ideology is, in relation to society, bureaucracy, medical independence, our responsibility to the community, and the crosscurrents of combat over "public" and "private" medicine is a help, not a hindrance. It is a practical matter, too—what is our final relation to authority? Do we serve the patient in a one-to-one human relationship? Or do we serve the hospital, the Army, the prison service, the PSRO, the FDA, the Blues or the Golden Calf? If your answer is "yes" to the first question and "no" to the second group of alternatives, then you are an anarchist, like Hippocrates, and you might as well get comfortable with the label. It has nothing to do with "right" and "left" or with communism and capitalism or with Tweedle-Rep. and Tweedle-Dem. It is something you do in the privacy of your office, not the hustings or the voting booth. Actually the lack of a label which cannot be misconstrued is one of the limitations on the vigorous force of American populism which believes in doing things yourself (direct action) with the cooperation of, and for the good of, others (mutual aid). Nor can you *vote* for an anarchist, because that would be a contradiction in terms—you vote for the authority which is the lesser evil. Listen to the debate at your County Medical Society, and count the number of speakers who would have a coherent view of medicine in society if they could bring themselves to call themselves anarchists, and you will see what I mean.

It is my earnest hope that when you have finished disagreeing with this book you will not necessarily write your own book, but ask your own questions about the nature of medicine and the nature of physicianhood. These are not the questions they ask us to test our fitness to be let loose on patients, but they are good questions nevertheless, and we need to answer them privately if not to others.

I

On Medicine

What Is a Doctor?

A physician is one who makes it his profession to take responsible charge of the treatment of the sick with a view, if possible, to cure or palliation. He, and with him I include the surgeon, is what the public refers to as a doctor.

It is interesting to ask what exactly a doctor is; it becomes necessary not only as the starting-point of a Socratic dialog, but for the practical reason today that some of his activities are about to be computerized. For this limited and auxiliary activity, which initially is all that is in hand, we need to analyze the task which is to be given to the machine. Clearly, if our appreciation of the nature of the task is incomplete, so will the machine's performance be. The majority both of doctors and non-doctors would traditionally agree that medicine is a unique activity—i.e., that in important respects it differs from other professional projects. One of these differences lies in the large component of unspoken, or transference-based, interaction which takes place between the parties to the medical transaction: doctor and patient. It might well be that on consideration, the unspoken and unconscious component in other mysteries, such as "pure" science, is equally important. But in medicine it is traditionally recognized, both from the history of the profession, which has its anthropological roots in shamanism—the expertise which deals with the interface between self and not-self (nature, sickness, guilt and expiation, the supernatural) and from the intuitive awareness among good doctors of the complexity of their own role and the profundity of the demands made on them by the patient.

This is traditionally expressed in Europe in the formula that medicine is an art as well as a science. That it is now (for the first time, in the last two centuries) fully a science is clear from the unwillingness most of us would feel at having our pneumonia treated by a charis-

9

matic physician with the knowledge of the year 1700. Patients today react with anger, spoken or unspoken, if they are told that the cause of their sickness is unknown and there is no specific science-based therapy for it. That medicine is an art is equally clear from the striking limitation in the effectiveness of scientifically hard-nosed but emotionally insensitive practitioners when dealing with common disorders. The need to write out this structure comes at a seasonable moment, when psychiatry is split between reductionist approaches ("this man is sick, whereas I, and we, are well, and we must cure him") and existential or Laingian approaches, exemplified by such writers as Szasz ("we are all of us sick, and I and society are equally involved in the failure of communication which makes us call this man mad").[1] It takes little philosophy to see that this bifurcation can be extended from the treatment of "insanity" to the treatment of broken legs. Medicine is observably split already between those doctors who see what the "existential" school is driving at—if only in terms of social medicine—and those who consider that the *only* treatment of a broken leg is to set it competently as a leg, not as a part of someone's body image and life-style.

One unique component of medicine is the experience involved in becoming a doctor. This is something which one important medical group, the lay psychoanalysts, do not share. It imposes both gains and deficits.

In the process of becoming a doctor, one begins, at an unripe age, with basic sciences. After a while, the student is introduced to death by way of the preserved cadaver. Soldiers and policemen are among the few groups beside doctors for whom human death, including their own, becomes tangible in their early 20s. The awareness of death becomes most intense in the post-mortem room, where the demonstration that people like us and of our age sicken and die becomes emotionally ineluctable. This experience may disturb some: others, more mature (and few of us are mature at the relevant age) are more upset by an intimate demonstration of the reality and multiplicity of human suffering. But the medical student soon finds that, though this man is incurably sick or dead, sickness and death can in many cases be dealt with, and it is his privilege to deal with them. The dragon is real enough, but the doctor is St. George, and he can really help—at least sometimes.

Doctors and Death

I do not want to go into the psychology of medical activism. As an armor against the intolerable it is needed by most of us, and at its best it becomes tempered down to a vigorous humaneness which we could probably get in no other way, and without which medicine would not be the same. Less desirable offshoots are the doctor's unease in the face of the uncurable; the leaving of the deathbed to the nursing staff (who are often religious and consequently not so bothered by death as we); and overt hostility to the chronic sick and the old. The point is that as a result of this experience the profession is moulded in a unique way, and if it includes scientists, those scientists differ experientially from their non-medical colleagues (many of whom are refugees into "hard fact" and the measurables in human life from the disturbing and the chaotic, of which death is the prime instance).

If I had one comment to make to psychotherapists who are not also physicians, it would be that they should not underrate this "existential" experience of being a medical student. They have a different experience—possibly equally stressful—at a different age. I can't discuss here, in the depth it deserves, the part which the awareness of death has played in human behavior. Enough to say that death is the subject which has replaced sexuality as the unmentionable thing in our culture. The Victorians, who were afraid of sexuality, had a large and overt experience of death. Loss of a parent was common, loss of a sib or a child universal. My generation did not have that experience. This may explain why it is prone to agree, if unconsciously, with Unamuno's idea of the tragic sense of life. The experience of death in war, which was perhaps our most characteristic experience of death, seems somehow different in its consequences on us from death within domesticity. I should declare an interest here—my research is concerned with the attempt to tamper biologically with the timing of age processes so as to control the human lifespan. I'm fully aware of the origins of that concern on my part—it springs from the experience I mentioned—but in fact I'm more concerned with the fact that it is a project in line with our society's expectations. Our generation has an acute intolerance of death, random or natural. Our children may well be, as Alan Harrington calls them, "immortalists"—Anglo-American culture is as intolerant towards acceptance of the present lifespan as Victorian culture became towards the acceptance of infectious diseases. When Prince Albert died of typhoid, the press described medicine as the withered arm of science. Within twenty years we had Lister, Pasteur, Ehrlich and Koch. The same is about to happen over natural aging, although the likely outcome is not the "immortality" of fantasy but a gain of 10 or 20 years of vigor, so that it takes 70 or 80 years to reach age 60.

Our attitude towards, and intolerance of, death are possibly more significant factors than ever before in shaping the experience we impose on medical students and nurses, and we ought to have enough insight into the social anthropology of our times to provide appropriate support—particularly if we wish to avoid the type of reaction formation I have mentioned. We may need something to put in its place. The shaman or medicine man, who is phylogenetically the oldest physician, has as his chief exploit or feat that he can harrow hell—that he can himself visit the dead, return unscathed, and sometimes, like Hercules, bring them back with him to life. This fantasy-exploit lies very deep in us, both as doctors and patients. We need to come to terms with it.

One way of doing so, which has been tried in Britain by Michael Balint[2] and others, is to initiate in-service training in psychotherapy—in other words, letting the students treat patients by psychotherapy under supervision from an early stage of their medical experience. The patients in general did very well, the students learned a number of skills, including that of handling transference and counter-transference without becoming armored or breezy, and an opportunity was provided for their own experience of mortality and of suffering to be verbalized, seen, and dealt with in discussion with the instructor. Significantly, when Balint's group tried to repeat this kind of insight-giving course with mature physicians, there was a 75 per cent dropout-rate.[3]

The physician in our culture, then, is often a man with a carapace. The carapace serves most of us well, unless we are disturbed or very thin-skinned, and it has served medicine for many years. Its inadequacy appears today only because the need to acquire the psychiatrist's different orientation puts a low valuation on paternalism and omnipotence. It is chiefly the psychiatrist who hammers into students the idea that their self-estimate must include awareness that there are patients who cannot be made magically happy, problem-free, and euphoric, either by drugs or interviews. Our fathers knew this, though they did not tell their patients. Our patients meanwhile give us every temptation to behave as gods or parents, or as wizards practicing black magic: it is only in the psychiatry course, where one exists, that students are explicitly taught how to handle these demands without harm to the patients or to themselves, and to handle them insightfully.

Another face of the physician, which we will have to consider carefully in writing our program, is that of the wizard or witch. The physician is not a wholly benign figure, any more than a parent or the goddess Kali is a wholly benign figure. He has his punitive and rejecting aspect, as the giver of prohibitions as well as boons, like God in the Hebrew Eden; and before we abandon that part of the unconscious machinery of transference we need to make sure that we can function without it. Adoption of this role is historically the second commonest form of medical acting-out—the creation of moralistic anxieties. The shaman nearly always reinforces his magic with a prohibition, and it is part of the natural history of medicine to do so.

The Computerized Doctor

One gets from a computer what one puts into it, and if one is to avoid stupid answers one must know what one is doing and phrase one's questions correctly. If we do not know what our business is about, the computer certainly does not. We are now on the verge of applying computers to medicine. Do we know what medicine is about?

It is relatively simple to use the machine as a textbook or a fund of experience. Here the physician codes and feeds in the presenting signs and symptoms, plus other relevant data. The machine will then either present the statistical probabilities of particular diagnoses, based on its "experience," or ask for more investigations, or both. It can jog the memory with key questions ("Does the patient work with lead?", "Is there any history of contact with rabid animals?"), it can ask with courteous persistence for the important piece of work you have skipped ("Is Kernig's sign positive?", "Have you done a rectal exam-ination?"), and finally it can inform you:

    Diagnosis: Emotional tension   95% Prob
              Migraine   4.55
              Brain tumor   < 0.05

leaving you to use your own judgment whether emotional tension and migraine are both present. Moreover, the machine can continuously update its own experience, provided you tell it the outcome in each case.

As a quick-reference checklist, fine. With refinement, we shall not need to type in the biochemical findings or the E.E.G.—given a suitable interface the machine can handle them directly. True it cannot handle subliminal knowledge, which is one of the physician's greatest resources—the pa-tient who "looks thyroid" or sounds schizophrenic, in the absence of any quantifiable physical sign—nor even the case which just seems wrong and rings an alarm bell in the mind. But it can be made to exercise an intuition of its own, based on the oddity of the inputs it is getting ("Have you considered symptom may be a delusion?").

So long as we use such machines to supplement our own experience, well and good. This is what textbooks are about, however, not what medicine is about. If doctors are to use computers more extensively, and in particular, if through avarice, inadvertence, or sheer work-load they start to use them substitutionally, we shall have a new kind of medicine, which is not closely related to our present practice. Medicine is not the diagnosis and cure of disease but the diagnosis and treatment of a patient who addresses himself to a physician. Now the diagnosis and treatment of a patient addressing himself to a machine, and limiting his contact with the physician to paying his bill, is a possibility. Some would say that in overloaded practices it is already an actuality.

When I was a student we were not taught to handle the communicative, non-mechanical part of medicine, but learned—if we had any aptitude—by watching good physicians at work. Most doctors now know from teaching what their ancestors learned by observation: that symptoms are messages, that patients come seeking not only relief, reassurance, permission, and treatment but punishment, purification, and even death or castration, and that now and again if the physician does not watch himself they may get what they seek. And here is the danger. The reductionist, scientific doctor (who is usually a little bothered by awareness that he too has emotions) is anxious to shed the anthropological side of his role altogether. If patients want shamans they should not. Disease is due to biochemistry, bacteria, immunology—whoever sectioned an emotional trauma?

This type of physician is the natural sucker for computer-medicine, or rather for its misuse. In fact, if he mechanized his practice, he would only transfer the shamanic role to the machine, which for our culture is ten times more magical than he is. All he will be missing is the opportunity to assume the real role which a physician can play through insight—a reconciler of biochemistry and of its emotional uses in the patient, of human hardware and software. If he does not, there is nobody left to do it, with art fragmented and priesthood unfashionable. Like the soft-centered physician (who recognizes that schizophrenia is a way of life but cannot admit that it may also have a chemistry, and who would not be seen dead using a computer because it insults the patient's personal freedom), he is missing out through lack of judgment.

Computer uses in diagnosis, and eventually in actual dialogue with the patient, raise the issue of existential versus reductionist medicine. This now is vocal chiefly among psychiatrists, but it applies just as much to broken legs or emphysema. And, as almost always in medicine, it is a matter of reconciliatory judgment, not outright confrontation.

I would rather see a relative of mine treated by a psychiatrist who had read both about Szasz and about serotonin than by one who, through his own personality difficulties, refused to entertain one or the other of these. It may well be that schizophrenia and autism have overriding biochemical bases, and that by restoring these we shall be able to set the schizophrenic in the same posture, vis-à-vis daily experience, as ordinary men. At the same time we shall not be abolishing the communication-defects in our families or our culture of which the schizophrenic is so devastatingly, and often so accurately, aware. Their ill-effects on him, on society, and on the doctor will continue to act to our hurt—just as air pollution will go on being a menace long after we find a short-cut cure for asthma.

I do not think it unjust to say that it is lack of judgment, not ignorance, which ensures that the two psychiatric schools continue to divide the subject (and that this judgment-lack is itself often a personality problem). The debate has not yet hit medicine, though all psychiatrists are aware it soon will. The point about computerized medicine is that it must not fall into the hands of the scientoid reductionists. Reductionists are, by reason of their innerly driven activism, brash and robust (they are the leucotomists of psychiatry): existentialists are often pathetically woolly and unaware of science. Consequently the patient, in his choice of counselor, is often at the mercy of the counselor's personality in the integrity of the advice he gets. A reductionist programming of a computer which was to substitute for the physician would only re-create the kind of half-physician which the reductionist often is. Yet even he, being a person, cannot quite cut out transference. He is highly effective with, though not very good for, the patient whose fantasy he fits, and who came to be treated rough.

On the other hand, since the design of a computer facility is often the work not of one man's unconscious but of a conscious committee, it might be easier to program one such in the direction of judgment than it is to educate judgment into human medical students. It is as easy to make a "straight" reference computer remind the physician of the emotional aspects of a syndrome as it is to make it ask him to do a rectal. In this respect alone, even if he does not know what to do next, the machine is educative.

Shamans and Oracles

But there is a far wider possibility.[4] It should eventually be possible to devise a mechanical system with which a patient could conduct a dialogue, as with a person—the difference being that, as in a mirror, the person with whom he talked would be himself. One could write an essay on the psychiatric importance of ordinary mirrors and of seeing one's body from an outside viewpoint. It is quite possible to envisage a system by which the patient may be enabled to see his mind from the outside, without the intervention of another person. True, for him there will be a "person" hidden inside the machine, taking various roles but in fact reflecting only the patient's own expectation (which is what, for much of the time, the human psychiatrist does). The machine, like the mirror, could (if we made it so) be neutral and reflecting—if the patient is hostile, it will type out WHY ARE YOU ANGRY? TRY TO TELL ME, and so on. Or we can make it directive, or explanatory (NOW YOU ARE ANGRY BECAUSE...). Or, better, we could make it sense which of these roles to play, in response to feedback from the patient and from its results in handling previous cases.

A mechanical or random system with which one can conduct a dialogue is called an oracle. In this respect the computer can do better in providing a "mirror" than did the oracular rods of the *I Ching* or the oaks of Dodona. It is odd that the primitive association of oracles with medicine, severed by science, may now be re-established usefully by technology.

Unless we do a great deal of discursive analysis of the unconscious machinery of medicine, our computer program, even when rudimentary, will incorporate our present hangups. If we do perform the analysis and leave the hangups out, we may find that because these are basic ingredients in a specialized and historically august form of human communication, worked out over centuries by trial and error, the hangupless model will work differently or not at all. In a sense we are already a mirror to our patients, and the unconscious preoccupations are mutual between us, or complementary.

We shall have to decide whether in reproducing medicine we leave out its warts, and whether any of those apparent warts are functional organs. What we certainly do not want—because it would not be that—is a fully "rationalistic" program for our machine: rationalism of that kind is itself an active and irrational denial of observable irrational forces. The kind of rationalism we do require is that which expounds those forces as exhaustively as possible, making them amenable to choice: whether our psychodynamics and anthropology are yet equal to doing this, to demythologizing medicine, I leave to you. It might in the event be better simply to let the machine reproduce our current prejudices—which are at least human and have been field-tested—and stick to white, or grey, magic, as good doctors intuitively do now.[5] But that will not dispose indefinitely of the salutary challenge posed by the machine—the need to understand what we are about. It may have to wait for a machine which is able to be non-discursively programmed, like a human mind—by observing its patients, or even by reading such non-discursive communications as myth or poetry. That machine would be virtually a psychiatrist, and a human-shaped one, because the preoccupations it would be scanning from its material would be archetypal, or at least common, human preoccupations. In fact, analog circuitry is uniquely well suited to scan allusive and nonparametric information of this kind.[6,7]

We have a start in that direction with structuralism as a form of analysis of human behavior. This interests both philosophers and anthropologists—the philosophers are interested to see what structures the human mind preferentially detects, and the anthropologists what structures in society reflect human thinking, language, and so on. This *is* the model of non-discursive communication between brain and society. If we had a pattern-detecting device in a black box we could unravel its store of exemplary comparison-patterns by seeing what patterns it detects when these are externally generated. The nice thing about our heads is that they are pattern-generators as well as pattern-analyzers, and they presumably use the same circuitry for generation and for analysis. This goes beyond the tautology that man and his works "fit" because each is adapted to the other. Freud's lifelong conviction that neurology would in the end supersede depth psychology looked much more naive ten years ago than it does now, although the outcome is likely to be a great deal more complex than the model he probably expected. At least it may supersede, or amplify, conventional philosophy and linguistics. If the program of the human mind cannot be read back discursively, that is only by reason of multiplicity or complication, not because it is in some way transcendental. Compared with the intuitive "fit" between communicating human beings, discursive printing-out is enormously uneconomic of time, and one could possibly instruct an analog machine without it if the machine drew directly on the patient's own software. But our culture is committed to the discursive mode and will never, I feel, be able to relax until it reaches at least some of the discursive answers. These will almost certainly coincide with the intuitive answers of medicine, but it will be nice to know that they do, and in arriving at them the machine's capacity to convert the analog and the allusive into the discursive and parametric mode may ultimately exceed our own—it may, in other words, take a machine to tell us how we function.

In the meantime, the attempt to use a machine as a doctor imposes on us a most useful discipline in examining all of the things which make up that role. What, then, *is* a doctor?

References

1. Szasz, T. The Manufacture of Madness. London, 1971.

2. Balint, M. Lancet ii:1015, 1957.

3. Balint, M., Balint, E., Gosling, R. and Hildebrand, P. Mutual Selection and the Evaluation of Results in a Training Programme for Family Doctors. London, 1966.

4. Spence, D.P. Human and computer attempts to decode symptom language. Psychosomat. Med. 32:615-626, 1970.

5. Day, G. Lancet i:211, 1962.

6. Chesler, L.G., Hershdorfer, A.M. and Lincoln, T.L. The use of information in clinical problem solving. Mathemat. Biosci. 8:83-108, 1970.

7. George, F. Government by computer. Sci. J. 5:76, 1969.

On Healing Americans

The concepts in this chapter were originally directed, not to psychiatrists, or future psychiatrists, but to medical students, internists, surgeons, pediatricians even, in the making. Psychiatry is in the process of recognizing the cultural determinants of healing—medicine among its wiser practitioners is concerned that its treatment may cure while its communication fails to heal. This concern, with its concomitant self-scrutiny, is predictably more difficult for the established physician. It needs to be addressed by all of us, early.

Psychiatry has a special role, nonetheless, in addressing the physician, and in overcoming resistances which he exemplifies. His attempts to understand the disaffection of his patients with scientism and their search for "holistic" medicine may prove a suitable point of entry. Teaching psychiatry to medical students involves not only the customary syllabus, but a consideration of what the physician is and does, or rather—in the face of attitudes which sometimes see medicine as a trade rather than a profession—what he should be and should do. If this sounds presumptuous, it is only the logical result of the pretensions of psychiatry, and the task should be undertaken.

George Bernard Shaw aggressively denied that *Mycobacterium tuberculosis* was the cause of tuberculous disease. To the extent that the disease does not occur in its absence, he was wrong. To the extent that the bacterium may be ingested without the taker contracting tuberculosis, he was right. Environmental, genetic, social and economic forces determine the individual's response to infection, and Shaw, as a social reformer, wished to focus attention on these forces. The bacteriologists, with equal justification, wished to identify the organism, and kill it when identified. Both were right, but in the main the weight of clinical practicality, as McKeown has shown,[1] has been on the side of Shaw, for the steady decline in tuberculosis began before the identification of the pathogen and long before the discovery of specific antibiotics against it.

Holistic Medicine

Holistic medicine (Gk holos, whole—the intrusive 'w' of popular writing is a solecism) presumably means that medicine which recognizes disease as involving several universes of discourse, or therapy as involving the "whole man," or both. Its antithesis, if it had one, would be not allopathy but the univocal models of medicine—pharmacotherapy, psychotherapy, surgery, and other single therapeutic techniques when elevated to the status of panaceas. Or more correctly, it would

19

be that medical orientation which founds its therapeutics on a single analogy—the body is a biochemical system, disease is a reflection of unconscious forces, and so on. Non-holistic medicine is in fact project-centered medicine, but one in which the tactical choice of priorities has been converted to a strategy, and the strategy, under cultural pressures, into an ideology.

It seems historically clear that the medicine which we now practice is project-centered. Both its projects—the control of infectious diseases and the making feasible of surgery, which depended on their control—and the strategies adopted to this end were set in the nineteenth century: bacteriology, immunology, chemotherapy and hygiene. Whether or not the enemies it recognized were already on the retreat, as McKeown suggests, is beside the point: the strategies were eminently successful, and for that reason the project, although it has not been fully completed, can now be seen as a project, whereas to our ancestors in the field it appeared to be a general philosophy of medicine. With the defeat of old enemies, new enemies, or rather equally old enemies who formerly stood in reserve, have taken their places. As Lalonde[2] points out, Canadians no longer die of smallpox or intestinal obstruction. Instead they die of tumors which have environmental, genetic and cultural determinants whatever their intracellular origin, of hypertension and cardiovascular disease, which appear to be largely cultural and dietary in origin, and a miscellany of causes (alcoholism, road accidents, suicide, gunshot wounds) which are indubitably consequences of life-style. Behind these stand in reserve the physical consequences of the process of senescence, which the majority of people in prosperous countries now live to reach. The only major sortie of medicine against the diseases of lifestyle and the self-destructive behaviors has been that of psychoanalysis, which focuses less on cultural than on individual unconscious forces in pathogenesis, and has proved clinically to be less beneficial than instructive. Apart from the relatively recent growth of scientific gerontology, which has yet no clinical payoff, we find ourselves without a forward-looking paradigm, developing better and more expensive forms of first aid for the diseases which now limit the individual, and finishing off the mopping-up operation of the former project.

The success of that project involved a concentration of viewpoint on the model of the body as a biochemical system. The gains in knowledge from this concentration require no demonstration; not the least has been the immense revolution in biology ending in the discovery and interpretation of the genetic code. Since these insights have come from the application—the first systematic application—of science and technology to medicine, the medicine of the project was of necessity scientific and technological. But the change of style from the medicine of intuition and ignorance has involved losses as well as gains. It was necessary for Pasteur to fight off a traditionalist opposition which pointed out, rightly, that all disease was multifactorial before he could identify a common factor, infection by organisms, which was accessible to clinical interference.

At the same time, the business of medicine is healing, not knowledge. To the extent that medicine is a science, it is an applied science, and while all knowledge is eventually of clinical relevance it has been frequently pointed out that the whole of molecular biology has not yet produced a single major therapeutic technique, in spite of its contributions to pathogenesis. In the flush of project-centered success, the unspoken model of the body as a biochemical-mechanical system has been accepted generally both by physicians and patients. The remedy of "sickness" is more technology, and "health" is pursued as one pursues the health of an automobile, by regular inspection and repair by technical experts. Health is "that state of well-being which is maintained by skilled adjustment, intervention and repair," and this is just such an example of a style arising from a strategy which "holistic" ideas question, both on grounds of adequacy and of cost effectiveness.

The human body and its ailments are in fact a rationally comprehensible system. In psychiatry, at least, most practitioners are aware that they can often best proceed intuitively, but this is not because cause and effect are abrogated or intelligibility absent in psychiatric communication—simply that to write out the process in plain language would be defeatingly lengthy, while allowing one's responses to shape intuitively on the patient's responses is both quick and accurate if the intuition is sound. One rapidly discovers whether or not one can do this: there is nothing irrational about the results.

Nor, of course, shall we get "holistic" medicine out of the mixture of magic and marshmallow which is sometimes set up in contrast to objectivizing medicine as defined by the Project. The real change has close parallels in other areas. Victorian medicine reflects the insights— of scientific predictability and manipulative intervention—which came from Newtonian mechanics and the machine: its industrial counterpart was mechanization. Modern medicine recognizes the mechanistic infrastructure, but also the override from homeostasis. Its models for this neuropsychiatric override are dynamic programming and systems theory, neither of them magical or irrational; its industrial counterpart is in computer science and automation.

To be "holistic" we do not need to be quacks, but we need to consider software as well as hardware. We use intuition in psychotherapy by virtue of similarity between our own software and the patient's. Older physicians talked sagely about "suggestion" and the influence of mind on body, and then stuck as far as possible to the objectively manipulable at a physical level. We have the much harder task of reading back the exact processes involved when software processes make disease occur or recur and when they operate to restore function. Objectivizing medicine, as devised to handle the Project, made the conscious and sensible choice of leaving out software effects to acquire comprehension of, and control over, the hardware. The diseases it initially attacked were all-or-none conditions like anthrax or smallpox. These often had evident economic or social determinants—which could be attacked by public health and a rising standard of social justice—but they were not greatly influenced by software effects such as self-image or life-styles. Nor was it much use talking about the effects of "meta-needs" on the maintenance of health when one was threatened by major infections which could be attacked by hygiene and immunization, or by surgical conditions which, though mechanically simple, were inoperable so long as infections could not be controlled. Acute appendicitis could play hell with any attempt to relate health to life-style—with wild cards at large, there was not much mileage in healthy living unattended by luck. Those stochastic conditions have now been largely removed. To remove the next layer, including chronic heart disease and the malignancies, we have to investigate software effects.

Modern "Healers"

Symptomatic of the need for a different orientation is the tendency for educated Californians, who of all people live in close proximity with technological medicine when they can afford its rising cost, to go to unorthodox "healers." Healing, as a traditional medical role, is a casualty of technology, because so much of it depends on intuitive communication at a nondiscursive level, and it is difficult to maintain both styles at once. Committed to scientism, we suspect intuition and the nondiscursive alike.

In fact, the unorthodox "healer" of today may operate at the wholly charismatic level, but more often he genuflects to science by substituting a science-shaped rationale. The particular system matters little in content—normally it involves a series of analogic statements omitting the words "as if" (our energy in experimental verification can readily obscure the fact that in conventional medicine we may regard, and encourage the patient to regard, the body as a man-made system which can be objectivized and treated as distinct from the vivid experience of "self" which is more or less fortuitously attached to it: we too are leaving out the words "as if, for some purposes"). The function of these arbitrary systems is to catch the attention, express dissent from the Establishment posture, and calm the patient educated in a discursive culture where explanation is sanitization. The "as if" statements refer less to verifiable somatic phenomena than to cultural and internal aspects of the patient's self-experience, and starting from them the "healer" imposes dietary or other ordeals, gives the healing permissions (to be angry, to dissent from authority, including medical authority, to be sick, to recover, to die), and finally, where he is effective, to direct attention away from the objectivization of the body and its disorders, and thereby to reorder the body image and the patient's perception of his social and individual self.

When "healing" is linked to established religion, this goal is addressed directly through the language of the religion in question. When it takes the form of mumbo-jumbo and quackery, the function of this is to demolish the ideology current in the culture—objectivization of the body and its treatment as a machine or an artifact is itself in anthropological terms a religion, meaning a system or style which delimits the bounds of identity as against the objective. If the "healer" today is a theorist, and a quack or antiscientific theorist at that, he is so chiefly as the mirror-image of project-oriented medicine and its limitations, rather as Shaw was perverse about the tubercle bacillus. This role is not, however, essential to the rationale of "healing," which is to reorder experience by operations on the social image and the body image. "Healers" in prescientific cultures, such as the Navajo experts studied by Bergman, do in fact have a theoretical basis for their therapeutics which differs little except in terminology from the theoretical basis of much psychiatry.[3] They have ritual to support them and a body of empirical experience contained in it, which enables them to manipulate both body-image and self-image through dances, psychodrama, kin participation, and visualizations such as sand-paintings.

The unorthodox "healer" in our own culture has to invent his rituals out of limited experience and his own possession or lack of intuitive skill. Hindu mysticism, another popular recourse for the medicated but unhealed person, which is now available in an emasculated and prepackaged form from spiritual supermarkets, originally set out as the project-oriented attempt to suppress the characteristic human sensation of objective and separate selfhood, substituting oceanic experience. To achieve this reliably, intensive efforts must be made to monitor and control processes normally not brought to consciousness, and finally to manipulate those involved in the experience of self, by methods closely similar to biofeedback. It was observed in the course of this project that bodily processes and health itself appeared to be manipulable in this way through operations on the body image, but traditional Hinduism, intent on the spiritual value of oceanic states, regarded these as mere magic tricks *(siddhi)* and a spinoff from the more important task of perceiving, through personal experience, the conditionality of our perceptions of time and of the objective. Our priorities in the face of this body of well-researched experience are likely to be different. The ability to manipulate the body by way of the body-image is the essence of "healing", an idea which figures little in Hinduism, and the ability to recognize the objectivism current in our culture as conditional might well be seen as a valuable by-product— one which could reorder our values fundamentally, and which, indeed, occasionally does so when obtained through the technological short-cut of psychedelic agents.

Our patients, however, go to unorthodox "healers", most of whom are a pale and often commercialized shadow of their shamanic ancestors, because they do not get healing from us. They get treatment from us, for which they are extremely grateful so far as it goes, but which in an increasingly anomic culture leaves them short on "health" as opposed to sickness management and exhortative hygiene. This is a relatively new development—our ancestors in medicine, from Ambroise Paré to Fothergill, Benjamin Rush and the 19th century family doctor were often highly proficient healers out of great therapeutic poverty. It is often difficult to get over to a class of young men and women, primed to the muzzle with blood electrolytes, the difference between healing and sickness-management. At one time it was picked up non-discursively from the great clinical teachers, but these are now in short supply among the multiple-choice answer papers. Quite a good way of overcoming blank incomprehension is to take them through the cases of Paré or Fothergill, and invite them to examine how they, with the resources now at their disposal, would have handled them, and how they would handle them now in a situation which deprived them of the laboratory, the modern dispensary and the intensive care unit. The experience is practical, in that one cannot count on these things in all contexts, unless one intends—some do—to take lifelong refuge in a teaching hospital. It also serves to generate the outlines of a medicine in which investigations are seen as confirmatory resources seconding a grasp of clinical natural history; in which active medications are not used as placebos nor self-limiting conditions officiously medicated, and such valuable resources as tomographic scanners are treated as heavy artillery to be sparingly unmasked rather than as the refuge of the lazy and the litigation-shy. From this salutary exercise in simplification students very often come to descry the outlines of a much leaner and less self-indulgent practice of sickness management, and some acquire a perception of the nature of healing itself. That they usually insist on describing this as psychotherapy as if psychotherapy were a specialty divorced from the practice, say, of surgery, matters little—provided that when in later practice they perform an oophorectomy or a hysterectomy they realize that discussion with the patient of her attitudes to her body and the changes to be brought about in it forms part of the operation, if that operation is to constitute the healing of a person rather than a manipulation analogous to the replacement of a muffler.

It was inherent in the project-oriented adoption of the scientific style, now hypertrophied, that intuitive skills should take a back seat. Holistic medicine is a lot easier when there are fewer mechanisms which are required to be memorized, since it is easier to see the wood when the trees do not have botanical names on which we shall be examined. At the same time, while we are obliged to guard against iatrogenic diseases produced by the careless discharge of live pharmacological ammunition, the quacks and charismatics, both civilized and pretechnical, quite often cure conditions which we cannot. Allowing for misdiagnoses, credulity, fraud, and hypes of every kind, tumors do occasionally respond to the laying-on of hands, and generalized arthritis does sometimes disappear at a revivalist service. Such events are rare, and even the devout sensibly limit the scope of spiritual healing. I remember passing the Cathedral at Lourdes and seeing a one-legged man walking briskly into it on crutches. "Un optimiste sans doute" said the French taxi-driver. Older physicians who were familiar with the effects of morale on immunology and who labeled them "suggestion" and privately saw no limits in sight to the therapeutic powers of that ill-defined entity were not as upset as our students would be at the notion of such cures. We know, after all, that it is possible to die through bewitchment, whether one is a believer in magic or not. I have seen a British patient fatally bewitched by a pathological report. Psychiatrists have long suspected, though they do not seem to have demonstrated prospectively, a correlation between the incidence and site of malignancies and mental processes. This is not surprising: after all, we now know that immune processes are under central control[4] and that immunosuppression can be effected as a conditioned reflex in unsuggestible laboratory rodents.[5]

There is ground in clinical impression as well as in folklore and the claims of quacks and the converted to believe that the process of "healing", when it successfully modifies the body image, can in fact heal, and can heal intractable conditions. Cautious attempts are now being made to verify statistically whether, how often, with what reliability, and under what circumstances, this occurs. There is no ground now, as there might have been when project-centered medicine was making its case and when George Bernard Shaw looked like a wrecker, to be nervous about such investigation. Of course every psychic, enthusiast and quack will rush in, as they are rushing into "holistic medicine", from acupuncture to pyramid energy. Yet the scientific method has taught us integrity of verification if it has taught us nothing else, and the lesson cannot be unlearned.

Nobody need be scared of a return to magic: that risk would only arise if we retreat into a scientism which itself is antiscientific. The value of verification is a necessary discipline which enables us to address even the oceanic experience of Hinduism and the conditionality of the objective without alarm if we keep our heads. If meditation cures tumors, that fact can be demonstrated statistically, and the sophistication of modern statistics is capable of dealing with arguments that failures result from lack of faith or the wrong attitude. Healing, as a reordering of the self, and the acceptance of responsibility for health, is not in its traditional form always curative. The healer's assignment includes reconciliation to death, which is an inevitable feature of the life cycle. At the same time, it may well have tappable resources to contribute to the control of disease. If it proves that meditation does cure cancer, we may of course opt for the quick fix, isolate the immunological or hypothalamic pathways involved, and look for something which we can administer by injection and market as a product. We probably should do so for the use of those whose meditations prove unproductive, but experience suggests that we shall be missing the distinction between the healer and the serviceman at an auto garage if we prefer that approach.

Healing and Treatment

However, spectacular interference with pathology by purely mental or attitudinal pathways, which is what the public expects of "healing", is not what is lacking from project-oriented medicine. It is another technique, if it works; and if it can be shown to work, the underlying religion of objectivism and manipulation as sources of "health" will be unshaken, because what occurs will be translated in short order into terms of oligopeptide hormones and central control of tissue reactions. This will be splendid, but is no more "holistic" than the discovery that resistance to smallpox is due to antibodies. Even if charismatic effects on pathology prove trifling or wholly fraudulent, enough is already known of biofeedback at the laboratory level to spark off an entire trajectory of research on cerebral control of cellular physiology. Only certain "healers" work by the production of instant sickness-control, and these tend to be either "saints" (meaning persons who impart insights going beyond the removal of disease) or Faustian figures who might just as well produce results by giving injections. Journeyman healers aim to produce the insight without the spectacular cures: Paré and Fothergill practiced medicine, not shamanism.

The difference between spectacular healers and healers is the same as between spectacular medical technicians and the physician. A far sounder model of "healing" than the instant or miraculous cure is found in the group therapy of terminal cancer patients[6]; here the objective is indeed healing rather than cure. The hero of *The Death of Ivan Ilyitch* was healed in the act of dying of his disease. If we overdefine this process, and say that healing consists in a collusive effort between doctor and patient which enables the patient to experience wholeness as wholeness, we are apt to run into the view that patients come for control of symptoms, not for edification, and that attempts by physicians to edify, whether by preachments or by psychotherapy, are already oversold—and tend in any event to come out of fortune cookies. Preachment has nothing to do with it; effective healing may include "psychotherapy" at a verbal level, but a great deal is nondiscursive and is communicated nonverbally, as every psychotherapist knows. Healing begins with the symptom, true, but its real difference from sickness management is that in addressing the symptom, whether we are able to remove it or not, we enable the patient to correct his internal phase relationships. Terminal patients in group therapy do in fact live longer, not because the opportunity to speak and to be heard arrests the disease, but because they fail to die prematurely from anger, frustration and despair. A meaningless and therefore frightening experience acquires shape; the members of the group and its rituals provide surrogates for the kin and the rituals which the Navajo use in like case, but which our culture lacks. If it proves that in some cases the disease itself regresses, that will be an uncovenanted benefit and an example of the other modality of healing.

A better example than terminal cancer, if the student wants to know the difference between healing and treatment, is the case of the individual with recurrent episodes of gastric ulcer and mounting hypertension. Treatment can suppress these; and stop the cycle surfacing elsewhere as alcoholism or an auto accident. Treatment plus healing will end the recurrence. The veterinary view of medicine will operate on the stomach and administer antihypertensive agents, both necessary measures. The enlightened practitioner may consider adding referral to a specialist psychotherapist by way of showing holistic-willing and recognizing the self-destructive inner "set" which is leading to the cycle of symptomatic disease. The healer will operate and prescribe, but will initiate the psychotherapy by the way in which he addresses the patient. At this level explanation, discussion and edification are less significant, if present at all, than his manner on entering the room and the fact of touching and being touched by the patient. This is why "healers" are born (or produced by direct infection from other healers) not made by taking notes.

We also need surgeons and diagnosticians, and the student—who is convinced from his technological background that anything can be learned from instruction if one applies oneself—may have to face up to the fact that being a healer is not his bag. Unless he can acquire the capacity nondiscursively he had probably better not try, and limit himself to realizing that the potential exists.

There are aspects of the process which can be learned or ritualized, however, and it is these which the inrush of technology has displaced. The oldtime medical student learned them because there was less factual instruction and technology to occupy his time, and he healed passably, however uncharismatic his approach. One can, after all, learn to play chess without being a master, and the fiddle without being Menuhin.

The Hippocratic rituals of history, examination, diagnosis, prognosis and treatment are all apt to the development of the skill of healing, or its subversion if ill conducted, for they can convey the manner in which the physician views his patient, and reinforce or modify the way in which the patient views his own condition. Medication is a powerful psychiatric instrument; the patient expects it, even if his condition is selflimiting, and his expectation indicates his view of symptomatology, which can range from excessive fortitude through suspicion of the medical resources he has invoked, all the way to projection of omnipotence on the physician. When I was in general practice, the patient expected, and the ritual of the culture prescribed, a bottle of medicine. The agents which this bottle contained were mildly active, but its function was that of a transitional object or talisman. Bearing the official stamp of the physician and the patient's name in a fair round hand, it was placed in the patient's home as a tangible evidence of the physician's concern, a permission to experience sickness without anxiety, a token of the doctor-patient relationship, to be ritually inspected and drawn upon three times a day; one tablespoon in water. Its existence spanned the period of therapeutic inactivity and observation during which selflimiting disease recovered, grave disease revealed itself, and the communication implicit in healing was set up.

Bottles of medicine no longer exist. Their place has been taken by highly active and often expensive medicaments with side effects. The student must become aware how frequently these scientoid prescriptions, often of mood-manipulating drugs such as the minor tranquillizers, are therapeutic rather to the doctor's sense of science than to the patient's condition: they may in fact withdraw our permission to experience it by rendering him tranquil.

At some time—and the coming to terms with the therapeutic role of observation and inactivity, and of the timescale of communication is as good a moment as any—the student needs to be discursively instructed about the meaning of countertransference. Who is to be made to feel better by the prescription, the physician or the patient? Should we invariably relieve a symptom, regardless of the unexplored situation of the patient vis-à-vis his body? Are you telling us to go back to gold pills and the placebo effect, and if not, what are you telling us? Are we not supposed to be scientists? No, you are not, you are supposed to be physicians who make use of scientific knowledge. Should we order investigations? Of course, if they will affect diagnosis, prognosis or treatment, and if you understand them and are confident that the clinical laboratory will produce meaningful results, and that you will fully understand the results when you get them—not otherwise, and not as a means of avoiding clinical examination and the formation of an overall preliminary diagnosis, certainly not to reinforce your own sense of power by role-playing the scientist. We all role-play, and you are supposed to be playing the role of physician-healer. At this point we shall need to alter both the gung-ho scientoid (there are only two sorts of cases—those you treat with specific medication and those whom you refer to a psychiatrist) and the amateur psychoanalyst—the first in full flight from the recognition and exigencies of human communication, the second intoxicated with the forces of the unconscious as some people are intoxicated with Shakespeare cyphers, numerology, or Biblical prophecy. Neither makes a good healer. And so it goes.

The intelligent student will reply that we are all emotionally involved in our roles, but the superego approves the rationalization and we can be careful not to act out—for which reason he prefers the detachment of science to the transmission of insight by nonverbal means. The brash will say "Countertransference, why? I'm going to be a gynecologist, not a shrink." In either case the proper answer is "Because if you don't recognize it, you will be a menace, scientific or otherwise, and instead of practicing healing intentionally you will practice black magic unintentionally." The dimension of communication cannot be turned off—either you use it to further the therapy or you use it to make things worse. As to the future gynecologist, he had better beware, for women are now not only more aware of their bodies and of inherent difficulty in communicating the experience of their body image to men—they are also highly sensitive to the attitudes which the gynecologist communicates. If these include sexual enthusiasm or hostility, or zeal to attack the anatomical symbols of motherhood and manipulate them, they will recognize this and let him know.

The insightless surgeon who communicates only with the anesthetized subject is next on the list, be he never so good a technician. One cannot explore the recesses of another person's body and remove important parts of it without communicating something—either one does it properly and heals, or one does it badly and bewitches, or one declines to communicate at all, sends an assistant to see the patient, and becomes a demonic rather than a human figure. People can be altered but not healed by a force of Nature personified. I know that surgeons have busy schedules, but the surgeon who does not include in his operating time the time to talk extensively to every patient communicates something to me if not to those he treats. A wizard is a demonic figure whose skills provide negative results to offset their brilliance. Etymologically he is one who is too "wise" for his own good, as a drunkard and a coward are too drunk or too cowed for their own good. Even the absence or invisibility of the surgeon, like the silences of the analyst, communicates something to the patient, and that something is nosogenic.

The same point—the difference between healing and treatment—can be made in another way, without reference to psychiatric terminology, if we prefer: students whose knowledge of their own difficulties in handling death, suffering, and communication makes them experience psychiatry as threatening can be introduced to Ryle's[7] concept of the natural history of disease. The naturalist is a scientist, in that he is an observer, but he is an observer with empathy for organisms in the wild state, recording and attempting to obtain an overview of their behaviors in an ecosystem. He observes real mice, which are organisms in a continuum of organisms, whereas the laboratory scientist observes lab mice, which are effectively artifacts of science, selected over years for survival divorced from mouse social behavior, weather cycles, pheromones, and dietary fluctuations. The healer is a naturalist who sees his patient as an ecosystem within a larger ecosystem of which the physician is a part. The scientoid sees him as a laboratory human possessing a body which contains a liver, in the enzymes of which the scientoid

specializes: placed in the consulting room, he does not sn
pop, he just lies there, and permits his tyrosine aminotran:
to be adjusted by a mechanic.

What is Healing?

The healer is a naturalist. Not all of us make good naturalists, and all
of us have unconscious motives. Our place may be in the laboratory or
the library, just as there are those whose only fulfilling place is the
monastery—they march to a different drummer. If students are frightened by the idea of all this and nonverbal communication too, let them
remember that they will have colleagues. One can be too shy or too
obsessed to heal by communication, and still be a dab hand at refixing
a torn retina or reassembling a badly smashed face. Let him then use
the skill he has, but see that the process of communication is dele-
gated. There was a brilliant urologist in Hollywood who so resembled
a gargoyle that he employed a physician of presence to front for him
and perform the interviews. Thus *clinical judgment may lie in knowing when one is not cut out to be a healer*—and in not trying to compensate for being tone-deaf by denying the value of music. The
student who reads Feinstein[8] will come away with the impression that
clinical judgment is something to do with the standard deviation of the
mean. It is rather the skill which is absent from any physician who
says that he advises this, that or the other *routinely,* or who fails to
note that while his treatments cure his communication invariably fails
to heal.

Are we now any nearer to understanding what healing is? We have
circled and recircled about it. It is a reordering, not of the patient's
"self," which as a neurological experience bordering on illusion cannot be "reordered," but of his sense of position and state in an ecosystem of which his actual body, his body image, other persons and
the physician are all a part. This reordering involves the unlearning of
learned behaviors, criticism of self-evident beliefs, permission to experience unwelcome emotions, and recognition of the parts of the ecosystem—"identity," inner processes, brain, body, environment—as both
continuous and nondifferent. If this sounds like heavy going, we can
be reassured that it need not be written out or discursively expressed
"in plain words"—a great deal of it cannot be, by reason of length—but
it can be experienced almost instantaneously after suitable preparation: which is why nondiscursive communication, such as a touch or a
gesture, are so much more effective than a lecture. Mary Baker Eddy
claimed to reorder our concept of health by lectures: the charismatic

healer does it by the laying-on of hands, and scientizes the experience as a transfer of "energy." What in fact passes is far more of the nature of information in the technical sense that a virus particle contains information; the preliminary rituals set the scene, the permission and the information effect the result sometimes reinforced by a few significant words.

None of this is as rarefied as it sounds. Take the recurrent victim of stress diseases. His "I" is not himself, but a hero who carries the goads of great ambition, the inner knowledge of the power to achieve, and the "sense of injured merit" which landed Milton's Lucifer in Hell. His world is not filled with people but with enemies to defeat, rivals to surpass, and stepping-stones to tread on. His goals are both pathetically slight for the effort involved (getting Jones' place on the Board, having a Mercedes and a million dollars, affording a more splendid wife than his brother demons) and chronically unrewarding when reached, so that they are reached almost unnoticed and left behind in pursuit of the next token reward. The culture being a machine for the ideological reinforcement of this scenario, it is constantly reinforced—what could be more normal and healthy? His body is on a par with his Mercedes—it needs to be reliable so that he can outsit and out-stud the omnipresent rivals, but that can be attained by regular servicing by a skilled mechanic. Its only drawback is that he cannot trade it in, but he will find a medical mechanic of a like compulsive cast who will connive at the role of maintenance engineer.

What are the options for healing? We can warn him to go slow, or his body may do so by providing a heart attack, but then we shall have to deal with the depression of Don Quixote who has found, not that the giants were windmills, but that he is unable to go on knocking them over. He will get his bypass operation—and go on the bottle or opt out of a cruel world. It would have been far better to get him sooner and turn him around, but unless there is some mechanical problem he will not go to the doctor at all. A psychical symptom such as achievement depression or impotency is more hopeful—it at least betokens the onset of questioning. We can provide him with an over-ambitious and rejecting parent to explain his style; that will give him someone to blame, but by adulthood his behaviors are long since functionally autonomous, however they were learned in the first place. We can analyze or lecture him if he will hold still for it—he will flounce out, though, like the patients described in Freud's account of "wild psychoanalysis"[9] he may come back later, when the gaps appear at middle-age crisis. A healer of stature (and Christ was known primarily among his contemporaries as such) could say to him with devastating effect "Son, your failures are forgiven you," or "Go away, sell all that junk, and give the money to someone who needs it." But few have the charisma to carry conviction.

But here he is, in your office, complaining of something minor—he has hurt his knee trying to beat a younger rival at tennis: no single achievement however trifling can be allowed to slip. To a scientoid he is a successful man with a bad knee, who wants a painkiller so that he can play again on Saturday. To a physician-naturalist he is over-hurried, overtense, overkeen to win on Saturday, and overanxious to avoid any further investigation: he wants his knee fixed, and what has that got to do with his personhood?

You can of course say nothing, make a note, and wait for him to come back with something major. You can, since he is in the office, say that it is a good opportunity for a checkup, to save his time, and take his blood pressure. If it is raised, you have the ground to insist on the need for further investigation, medicate, and take time to establish the communication you will need. If you trust your charismatic ability, you can ask directly "Why is it so important to win on Saturday?" but that is your decision. At least high blood pressure is something he understands, a nuisance suggesting that a skilled mechanic was needed. If you are a physician-naturalist the entire communication of the background can take place in the first two minutes of the interview, without any verbal reference to any subject except knee, tennis and waste of time. If you in turn signal deference to the culture-image of success, you are colluding, not healing—if you signal resentment at it, he won't follow your advice. What you ought to signal cannot be learned, any more than you can learn to write good loveletters out of the letter-writer's guide. Either you will do the right—or the wrong—thing naturally, or you will learn by watching a natural physician, or you will serve as an efficient pit-crew and pick up the pieces when this patient crashes. You have some charisma going for you in that you are "the doctor," and a figure with whom he does not have to compete—perhaps a parent reminiscence he has to appease, although that too can make problems. Not being able to say "Son, your declining skills at tennis are forgiven you," you are going to have to take time, deal with noncompliance, and pray patiently for some other opening—a psycho-sexual problem to match the slipping tennis game, for example, to enable the can of worms to be opened, either by you or by a psychotherapist. But the eventual limits on the healing which will be achieved can be set in the first moments of the first interview.

The Making of A Physician

America—which almost alone among civilized countries does not have one—is in the throes of providing itself with a "health service."

Although what it may well get is a system of extremely expensive sickness management, which would be better than nothing, the very tardiness provides at least the theoretical opportunity of producing, alone among civilized countries, a genuine health service. This would involve by its nature the simplification of medicine, the sharing of responsibility for personal health between the doctor (professional) and the patient (nonprofessional), the reservation of auto garage Medicine for the functions in which it is appropriate, and the reduction of the need for specific intervention by a far greater education both of doctor and of patient. Holistic propagandists would like to make Tantrik yoga and consciousness-raising chargeable to Medicare—which would simply multiply rackets. This presupposes the ineducability of physicians. I do not think physicians are ineducable, though some have not had the opportunity as students to view the practice of medicine in its humanistic context, nor could they do so without some assisted work on their own attitudes to the profession they practice. One would be better off with a lay healer than no healer, but it seems unenterprising of the profession to leave healing to naturals and potential quacks—there is enough qualified quackery without buying more and unqualified.

What this means is that medical education has to enter the long road—traumatic for many teachers already grown old in scientism—of making self-examination and the acceptance of human skills a part of the medical curriculum, if possible arriving at a humanistic view of health and sickness ahead of, not behind, the cultural climate and the public at large. This may involve a certain selection between communicators and non-communicators, a certain amount of channeling, but no more so than in present channelings involving delicate surgery and manual dexterity, or biochemistry and mathematics.

Physicians and dentists in California have by far the worst accident record as civil fliers. Asked for his comment on this statistic, the flying instructor at Ontario airport said "Right: did you ever try to *tell* a doctor anything?" Aside from wincing, an appropriate reaction would be to devise a medical education producing doctors who did not need, in the matter of profound or hurtful subjects, to be "told" because they perceive. Such people are not scientoids or speculative tradesmen, but physicians. If this insight should overflow into the idea—terrifying, it seems, to many Americans—that society might become social rather than competitive and concerned rather than commercial, we might accept in the interest of health a reordering which we reject in the interest of social justice. But that is another story.

References

1. McKeown, T. Medical History and Medical Care. Oxford, University Press, 1971.

2. Lalonde, M. A New Perspective on the Health of Canadians. Ottawa, Government of Canada, 1974.

3. Bergman, R.L. A school for medicine men. Am. J. Psychiat. 130:663-666, 1973.

4. Ader, R., Cohen, N. Behaviorally conditioned immunosuppression. Psychosomat. Med. 37:333-340, 1975.

5. Stein, M., Schiavi, R., Camerino, M. Influence of brain and behavior on the immune system. Science 191:435-440, 1976.

6. Yalom, I. Existential factors in group therapy. Strecker-Monogr. 11, Pennsylvania Hospital, 1974.

7. Ryle, J. The Natural History of Disease. Oxford, University Press, 1939.

8. Feinstein, A.R. Clinical Judgment. Baltimore, Williams and Wilkins, 1967.

9. Freud, S. On "wild" psychoanalysis. Collected Papers, XI, 209, 1910.

The Limits of Medicine
A Commencement Address

You ladies and gentlemen who have the privilege, and are undergoing the ordeals, of being medical students today are about to enter the profession of medicine. This is an interesting and exacting time in which to do so, and not only because of the vast amount of examinable knowledge which will be required from your hands.

Medicine today is under criticism, some of it valid, some of it foolish. Considering the fact that most of us who are in practice are fully occupied with what Bacon called "the sordidnesse of Cures," and have not too much time for either philosophy or militancy, the profession's record of self-examination is—for a powerful and self-maintaining élite such as physicians—not bad. Young American doctors in particular have become increasingly disillusioned and dissatisfied with the growth of a massive, sometimes unscrupulous, and quite generally uncompassionate sickness industry—the medical Mafia, the cash-in-advance syndrome, the hospital real estate management tie-up, etc. We are living in a time when America, the only major civilized country without a proper health service, is being forced into adopting one. That lack could be an opportunity. Americans could import the British, the Canadian, the Soviet, the Swedish, the Dutch, or some other pattern—in that case they would have a fair sickness management service representing the philosophy and thinking of the 1960's. They can hardly import any such and get a *good* health service, for systems such as these on their home turf are the product of other societies. Europe's excellent health services, for example, depend on an attitude towards social service which is uniquely European. Americans could equally well start from the top and develop a true health service—nobody has ever done that yet—linked to neighborhood action groups and avoiding both the Scylla of cash capitalism and the Charybdis of Federal and local bureaucracy. The choice is theirs. I am of course a foreigner in America, but like all physicians, deeply interested in civil rights—the right of the individual to health care, the right of the doctor to practice without outside interference, the right to know, the right to confidentiality, and the right to human dignity in situations of sickness and death.

All of these are urgent practical matters, but at the same time the philosophy of medicine is not so much changing as becoming explicit. Good doctors in all times have combined what they had then of scientific medicine with the shamanic skills of the spiritual healer. They did and taught this intuitively—medicine is an art and a science: now through anthropology, not least the anthropology of the profession, we are coming to do it discursively. We recognize that science is necessary—if we did not have it, some 10 to 20 per cent of those here would already be dead. We also recognize that the scientism taught in some schools is a reaction-formation against self-knowledge and the difficulty of having to connect with people. Ivan Illich has pointed to the mutual deformation of medicine and the culture, which he sees as Faustian. Faustianism is very much what the anthropologist calls sorcery: the activity is neurotic and the result self-defeating.

Now the answer to Faust is not medievalism but Promethean humanism. We will never in all likelihood conquer death, but it is Promethean, and a task of medicine to try, so long as we do it with insight.

Hippocratic medicine has an anarchism of its own, in spite of the profession's conservative political image. Any medicine which owes its primary responsibility to anyone other than the patient—a government, employer, army, insurance company, or whatever, is not medicine but veterinary surgery. These are among the matters to which we ought to address ourselves. Another is the gross economic inequity of the distribution of medical care worldwide. This concerns me most of all—oddly it seems to concern the more extreme medical populists who also argue that medicine is a scourge which should be put down, and a cause of most of our illnesses—I'm not quite clear how they square the two. We do owe it to them, however, to look sensibly at iatrogenic disease: they have a point, particularly in regard to the unspoken creation of fears, expectations, and altered body awareness by involuntary medical shamans whose magic turns black. In the same context we must address the anthropology of nursing: the mother-father-child triad has always been traditionally recreated in patient care, or was until it was replaced by the intensive care unit with masked and anonymous psychopomps who are equally powerful as magical figures but somewhat different.

One has both to sympathize with and to envy the medical student today. One must sympathize with the killing pace of academic competition, the immense amount of fact which has to be learned without the concurrent stimulus of direct responsibility to patients which helps the physician to study and perfect his skills....with the pressures of society, which bear on all of us, but can, in your case, end by sapping ideals which you had on entering medicine....with the confusion generated in any student responsive enough to see beyond his or her nose by the babel of fashionable fads, some of them good in parts, others merely diversionary. It was easier in the 18th century when doctors knew less, had fewer skills at their command, learned by apprenticeship, and lived in what they (wrongly) believed was a stable social order. One has to envy you, in spite of all this, for the fact of living in times when change is imminent, since the nature of that change will be in your hands insofar as the practice of medicine is concerned. Oliver Wendell Holmes defined the Law as "what the Courts will actually do." We could define medicine in a given period in terms of how physicians actually practice; so how you will practice, since that will lie in your hands, makes you partakers in defining the posture of the profession.

Any intelligent American medical student who attends his county medical society on one of its political nights will see that in the face of these considerations American medicine, in its organized manifestations, is running hither and thither like sheep without a shepherd. It is intensely distrustful of a "health service" involving Federal finance (and God knows, if it were to be run by the GSA, the FDA or the mental like of the Department of Energy, who could blame it?). Anxious to keep its independence of judgment, harassed by a handful of bell-wethers who are more concerned with their pocketbooks than their patients, but unhappy about the loss of the godlike image which (it believes) the profession had in the past, it would listen gladly to any prophet who now arose to say, "Look, fellows, I have a better idea." As to the godlike image, I don't think most of us ever had one—we were doing a job we greatly enjoyed to the best of our ability, and we were unaffected by the pretensions of Dr. Kildare, the medical cowboy. It is the Doctor Kildares who swell the ranks of physician suicide and addiction—being such is an unenviable fantasy, and one would like to see it replaced by medicine done because doctoring is worthwhile and we enjoy it.

What we have seen is far more than a backlash against over-zealous technology or hucksterism. It is part of a coming cultural revolution including, but not confined to, medicine. The medicine which it forecasts is not new—rather it is the restitution of medicine in its traditional and Hippocratic role, free from commercial deformations and from the distorting effects of three dangerous modern illusions, the elitist expert, the crash program and the technological fix.

The future of medicine is to a large degree the future of society. If society is *dirigiste,* medicine will be directive. If we are on the verge of a period of war between embattled haves and a majority of have-nots, medicine will be a commercial luxury, and the same principles of greed and class selfishness will apply within nations as between them.

But if we are on the verge of a revolution as yet unclear—not a conventional or a nineteenth century Marxist revolution but a change toward ecology, ungovernability, regionalism without chauvinism, the devaluation of government, the valuation of the individual and the growth of neighborhood action, then medicine will change as part of that revolution. Nobody living in 1750 could have foreseen the nineteenth century, although they could have foreseen that the world would shortly look and feel different to those living in it. The cultural revolution and the social revolution are simultaneous and fuel each other. As our world changes, away from the world of technological and political paranoia—the term which perhaps best characterizes what we have now—to the world of post-technical anarchohumanism (Jonas Salk's "epoch B society") medicine will change in step, and I think Ivan Illich, as a Savonarola of the stethoscope, has rightly pointed to some, though not all, of the ways in which it will change.

Papers now appear lauding the Chinese as innovators. By all accounts they are, from their own political standpoint, running a unique new solution to the problem and ideology of health care which is different from the American commercialist, the European social-democratic-socialist, and the Soviet bureaucratic models. One would like to hear about it. We need all the data we can get if only to avoid other folk's errors. As it is, we have limited access, not so much to the administrative facts (China, in fact, has no overall health service: each commune runs its own) as to the totally Chinese and unexportable background on which such a service rests.

American medicine of the future may well be decentralist, too. It will also probably be simpler, if only on grounds of cost, and clinical skills may replace high technology. Noninvasive cardiologists have rediscovered the stethoscope, and—surprise, surprise—one can make diagnoses with it, using more complicated technology for checkup and backup. It need not bother overmuch about being vociferously "holistic"—good medicine deals in wholes, in prevention, and in the natural history of man by its own proper motion and without cult exaggerations. Our medicine will not be Chinese; it will be the medicine of a disorderly, acquisitive, but basically libertarian populist democracy which is in the process of being cut down to size by its own centrifugal forces and its inability to generate a coherent political expression of care for others, or find a substitute for Jolly Millerism ("I care for nobody, no, not I, for nobody cares for me"). It is also a society which, without meaning it, has exposed the play-therapy character of government, and has run into the problem of psychopathology in office—just as Soviet Marxism has done but in a different, American form: Nixon has slain his thousands and Stalin his ten-thousands, and neither one has reached the ostensible goals of the exercise.

This is the question which would probably be the first to be asked by a visiting martian psychiatrist—why do we give the lower decisions in research and technology to people of the highest ability, and often of disinterested integrity, but entrust our longterm planning, our priorities and our societies in general to psychopaths intent on irrational forms of play-therapy? I will not answer that question, but it is critical, and we have to answer it. In the pursuit of power, the pursuit of wealth, and the pursuit of conformity are irrationalities of this kind; where these conflict with teleonomic aims like health or even human survival, it is not the Leonardos, the Galileos, the Illiches, or even the populist majority but the people seeking office, who become what William Blake called "something else besides human life," who now make the decisions. Which side are we ourselves on?

If we look at medicine in general, I think it is already trended away from its past commodity and technology image by the logic of its research future. Some of the most promising innovations in medical technique already involve active patient self-help in a social setting—group therapy, the psychotherapeutic community and social learning experiences such as assertion training in psychiatry; biofeedback and operant conditioning for the control of autonomic processes in the field of therapeutics. This, if we can develop it, promises a technology of medical self-control which has the potential of substituting very widely for drugs in the management of conditions such as epilepsy, and in sociogenic problems like hypertension and anxiety—precisely the kind of symptoms where overmedication now obtains. In my own field, which is gerontology, we are looking at the possibility that some of these techniques can be applied to the treatment and control of aging: it would be ironic if this turned out to be the case, because then George Bernard Shaw, who long since made most of Ivan Illich's points about medicine, would be proved right about Methuselah, too.

These changes also involve a new kind of doctor. When we train physicians now in human skills like sex counseling, we have to make some of them over completely from the gung-ho, dirigiste mentality inculcated by the scientism of the last generation: Some—the good ones—are loving it; others, who got into science or money-making as an escape from self-knowledge, freak out or flip. The President of the American Medical Association can still pound on the desk and say he won't have the Government financing his competition, but people who talk like tradesmen get treated as tradesmen, and there is a new generation of American doctors who spend their time in the free clinics and who have regained the old joy of practicing on the sharp end of medicine which the office specialist has lacked. Change is, accordingly, on the way. I think that the criticisms we have heard, even if some of them are exaggerated, are a help rather than a hindrance—I am quite sure Illich will get read in medical schools, off duty if not in class. Many young doctors are already entering the free clinic movement. I think they and their colleagues, worker-priests of medicine, are the first of many. My old anarchist friend John Hewetson has practiced as a physician-activist for many years now, and his example is catching on. To do this properly one does not have to be a radical, but it helps. The essence of active health care does not lie in downgrading the doctor, but rather in upgrading the patient to the status of an equal partner in his own cure, but this upgrading is in itself radicalizing, since to cure ourselves we have at some point to confront and alter society.

I think in the context of the times we can all understand the going rate of disillusion with the application of technology to health, though I doubt if Pasteur or Ehrlich would have understood it. We do well to criticize, but we need to remember that we are criticizing from the position of beneficiaries who take technology for granted.

As in all American contexts, our Fundamentalist evangelical ancestry is not far below the surface. Already we meet patients who believe that most if not all medication is suspect. If we give active drugs as placebos and diagnose diazepam deficiency in every anxious American, they certainly have a case. The pharmaceutical industry is under a cloud with liberated public opinion.

We have heard the pro's and con's of pharmaceuticals. My own attitude here, I think, is best exemplified by two experiences from when I was a medical student. I can remember a man who was dying of subacute bacterial endocarditis. He was a great guy, it was a very sad case, the lesion was so simple—we all went in a body to the Professor and asked: "Isn't there some way to get at this?" There wasn't, and he died. A few months later we got our first penicillin. That patient just missed the bus. This disease is no longer fatal—it can be dealt with by antibiotics and open-heart surgery. On the other side, we used to see dozens of cases of so-called pink disease in infants; these, it later proved, were due wholly and entirely to mercury in teething powders. When I was a child they used to grind up mercury with chalk and give it to me, which is very probably why (in the opinion of colleagues who disagree with me) I am crazy now. Long after this was known, pressure was still being put on the manufacturers to take these infernal things off the market. The manufacturers, a small firm, simply didn't give a damn.

Pharmacology itself is an ally if we use it properly, and there is no point in bad-mouthing it indiscriminately. The best way to control atheroma is by diet and exercise, but we would all welcome a drug which prevented it. The work of Finch at the University of Southern California indicated that the depression of old age is linked to catecholamine changes—it can be modified by antidepressants: at the same time being old in America is a depressing business and we need social militancy—such as that of the so-called Grey Panthers—to make it less so. Both aging in some of its aspects and cancer may well become accessible to immunological attack before long—this will create a potentially difficult priority question if the method is tailormade and therefore expensive, but it would be foolish not to develop and use it. The enemy is really over-treatment with ineffective, harmful or unnecessary drugs which are ordered out of laziness or for lack of more appropriate symbols of caring and support.

What are the conclusions we can properly draw?

1) Because in rich countries medicine has been treated as a commodity, rich people are over-medicated to their hurt, and poor people, though not over-medicated, are medicated (if at all) to keep them quiet. Drugs are used (as they always have been) not only as specifics—the leading achievement of modern therapeutics—but also as placebos or as symbols. But those we now use, unlike the ground bark and the woodpecker beaks of the witch-doctor, are active pharmaceuticals and can be abused.

2) Social anomie, the lack of appropriate rituals, and the lack of family, have laid on the physician a number of demands which really are reconcilable with sickness care only if the physician fully resumes the role of shaman or medicine man, and shamanism is hard to reconcile with so-called rational medicine. Accordingly, the doctor has tried to deal with human matters like birth and death through technology, and the result is an incompatible mixture.

3) Rising expectation has led to the idea that technological medicine can deal not only with illness but also with stress and unhappiness. It can't, and it should not try.

4) The limits of technological medicine need no external definition because it is already too unwieldy to last. Medicine is changing and our own epoch must make the change. In essence it is a change towards better judgment—not a doctrinaire rejection of drugs and technology—simply an end to their foolish, exploitive and uncritical use.

5) Power structures, whether governmental or commercial, will always try to abuse medicine in order to control and institutionalize

people, as they abuse everything else. The governmental paradigm of the good society is a progressive prison. The commercial model is a well-run version of Las Vegas. Through inadvertence and involvement in the society in which it works, medicine has sometimes gone along with these paradigms: commercial sickness industries in capitalist countries, the existence of psychiatric police directed against dissidents in both capitalist and communist countries. Someone has to make medicine more aware of these abuses, and get it back where it should be, on the side of the patient and not the status quo. True medicine is our oldest anarchist institution. It puts the individual first: if it isn't anarchist, it isn't medicine.

6) Doctor and patient aren't father and child or God and worshipper. They are equal partners in the adventure of healing, where transference and counter-transference are of equal importance. Nothing else will work at the all-important human level. It is not base or unnatural to need consolation. We need to get it from our fellows, doctors not excepted, and it has its place in a true medicine. If we had a humane society we could give it to one another. Much of what is being treated now is not illness or dysfunction but lack of a feeling of personal well-being.

The therapy for that disorder is a change in society. For some complex reason, it is traditional that the physician be most often a conservative by opinion, and that the conservative enter medicine. There are in medicine and in society conservatisms which are right and humane. But where society and its ways are pathogenic, there is also an obligation on the physician to advocate and demand change militantly, if necessary, to prescribe it for his patients and to adopt it in himself. I have said that the physician is an anarchist and it is a belief of anarchism that the revolution begins in yourself before it begins in society. The doctor is well placed, if he wishes, to resist both commercialism and bureaucracy, both callous laissez-faire and the manipulative abuse of medicine, psychiatry and surgery as control mechanisms— he has an august tradition of doing so, ever since flogging in the British Army was dropped because physicians refused to continue to supervise it.

All I can say is that I wish I were now entering the profession as a student again so as to have a hand in the coming fight.

And yet, as one soon discovers, it is quite false to depict the process of change as a battle. That is not how it is experienced most of the time. The belief that it should be so experienced is the leading error of romantic revolutionists, who get their battle and do with it more harm than good. The proportion of overt conflict in useful social change is about 1 or 2 per cent—the rest is prosaic, practical activity. If it gets higher than that, we start spawning our own demagogues.

One of the main reasons that doctors are an effective force for change if they wish to be is that they have no time—assuming them to *be* doctors, not medical politicians on the way up—to strike ideological attitudes. They have to treat patients. But in a free society, in the course of ensuring that their patients are treated, or can afford to be treated, and will not have the gains of treatment dissipated by non-medical forces such as poverty, war, and chronic insecurity, we find ourselves social activists not by choice but simply as part of the job in hand. The most revolutionary task any of us are likely to have to undertake in a democracy is the devising and setting on foot of care delivery systems which we ourselves operate, with our colleagues and patients. What is revolutionary about that? Well, simply that we ourselves have to put them in place, not look to others to legislate them. Some of their features, if they are well-conceived, may indeed be legislated afterwards, but that is a by-product. It is also, in my view of medicine, the right way around. Moreover, it is purposive—cutting out the play-therapists—and it is democratic in the true sense, in that it comes about in concert with our own local community, admits diversity, and permits choice. It also lays very heavy responsibilities on us and on our standards: much, much easier to buy a package, to rely on benevolent centralism, or simply to operate the system as we find it.

I can remember when British hospitals for the old were warehouses, and those who sought jobs in them were the lazy, the impaired and the failed among physicians. A relatively small group of individuals—none of them an ideological militant—turned some of those rookeries into model geriatric centers which attract medical tourists worldwide. They did it not by making speeches or seeking social battles, but by practicing good medicine—the 1 to 2 per cent of combat arose when that practice was frustrated administratively or fiscally, and the combat was successful chiefly because the combatants were manifestly disinterested and doing an excellent job. You cannot legislate a "health service" other than permissively but you can create one; and if it is created locally and and in variety it will offer a choice of tested options for wider adoption. Americans often think of the British health service as a socialistic imposition: it was indeed set up by a social-democratic government, but what was done was really the institutional consolidation of family practice. Family practice in turn was the institutionalization of medicine as it had grown up in a society based on the village.

Now America, in addressing what it will eventually choose to institutionalize, has neither of these traditions. To institutionalize primarily the medicine of the hospital and the specialist would, in my view, be a cardinal error—one which its astronomical expense may fortunately prevent. What should be institutionalized is up to you, the physicians, and your patients to explore jointly. It is precisely because neither the public, nor the profession, nor Washington has any clear idea what should be institutionalized to form a "genuinely American system of health care" that local experiment becomes so challenging. That is the view from the hilltop of graduation these days: the new graduates shake hands, disperse, some of them into academia or specialism, but a growing number into the general landscape of primary care where these problems are to be addressed and the skills of the physician as the architect of change will be tested. There has probably been no time since the Founding Fathers when the chance for the construction of basically novel and humane social institutions simply by doing one's ordinary, daily work has been so good. And in wishing you well, I think it is that prospect which I envy you. You are going to find out what the limits of medicine really are.

II
On Psychiatry
Psychiatry and Happiness

People have traditionally consulted the doctor because they were ill. It is a relatively new development that they should consult a doctor because they are unhappy. We now demand the right to health: in contrast to his forebears, the man for whose condition there is no specific therapy is inclined to be disgruntled (what is science for?). The right to be made happy is a newer demand.

It is not altogether insightless. Pathological melancholy has always been seen as a disease, by doctor and patient. One of the most important clinical facts to get over to the student is the commonness of mild depressive states presenting in various disguises. Severer depression is a medical emergency and its immediate relief a medical problem: the insightful depressive goes straight to the doctor—the less insightful, whatever the chief preoccupation worrying him, is more and more likely to be sent to the doctor by his priest or bank manager, as public awareness about affective disorders spreads. In fact we can go too far in that direction, and forget that people really may go mad for grief, love or mortification—yet even for the primarily reactive state, since we cannot shoot the patient's relatives or rivals nor restore the dead to life, medicine comes first and psychiatry or reconciliation often second. Even classical depressive psychoses, which respond to drugs or ECT, are usually triggered by something.

Counseling

It is not the suicidally or lethargically unhappy patient who sets our main problem in regard to happiness—it is still not clear how much of his reaction to circumstance is biochemical and constitutional. All of the growing volume of psychiatric counseling is directed to the unhappy by definition. But as a matter of fact we shall not expect, if we have any insight and are not under the influence of medical feelings of omnipotence directed to making *ourselves* feel happy, that counseling or even full analysis will take unhappiness away. Much more of our time will actually be devoted to enabling people to admit and experience feelings of loss, grief, anger and frustration which their personalities, and modern town culture, have not equipped them to deal with. Many if not most of the physical conditions which appear in the GP's office are at some point substitutes for the toleration of unpleasant emotions. Psychiatry is less concerned with making us permanently and fatuously euphoric than with making us sufficiently strong and adult to tolerate being occasionally, or even frequently, otherwise.

Human Communication

One obviously can and should dispense reassurance and consolation where possible; this is merely human communication. The patient's demands, however stoical he looks, will always go beyond this; even for the hardiest subject, the doctor is a parent who will "make it well." He may delude himself into playing this rôle, and in any case he may be wise to accept it temporarily to give the patient something to lean on—regression for a while, whether into swearing or into dependence— is a safety valve. The long-term aim is to substitute adult toleration of the real buffets of life, and the willingness to accept grief, for neurotic anxieties or their physical and reactive offshoots. This includes the re-experiencing and admission to consciousness of sorrows past and no longer relevant, and ultimately the acceptance of our total experience, both of ourselves and of the world. At the moment we barely allow ourselves to experience bereavement.

Medicine gets this task today because society offers so little in this direction. It has none of the elaborate and sophisticated emotional technology we find in so-called primitives which deals intuitively and socially with unbiddable drives and emotions by ritualization, symbolism, and various types of psychodrama and of abreaction. One might have commended this lack in our world to a recent editorialist who argued on statistical grounds that the World Cup was a bad way of ascertaining the most competent football team: an anthropologist would see it as one of our few surviving ritual conflicts and a minor safety valve for aggression, which is one of the parts of ourselves that a humane and civilized ethos finds hardest to accept. The violence of our entertainment may possibly be another. By witnessing the shedding of ketchup we possibly avoid not only shedding blood (though we do too much of that), but also taking out our feelings on public property or our own stomach wall.

In our assessment of the psychiatric importance of happiness we may have been misled semantically by Freud's apparent hedonism. This now looks naive, in terms of animal study: animals, including ourselves and our infant selves, are probably not propelled by a search for sensory satisfaction *per se*, which was the old Freudian formulation, but by a search for minimal tension. Wanting food when we are not hungry, or sex when we have just had sex, are typical displacement activities where the apparent aim is covering-up for some other tension. The ideal equilibrium is not constant libidinal satisfaction, nor even a Buddhist absence of sensory interest, but a balancing-out of tensions at a level which is tolerable and compatible with wellbeing. The Buddhist non-involvement recipe itself involves tension—or would, if it were attainable in good faith—with our desire for activity.

If happiness meant total wish-fulfillment, ranging from absolute control over the demands made by our fellows to personal immortality, man would indeed be an unhappy organism. On the other hand, if he got this, he would stop being Man. Adult humanness rather than superficial happiness is the aim in view, and it is this which psychiatry (and society) ought to foster.

Research on Drugs

Where unhappiness is overwhelming, whether in anxiety, depression, or the confusion of the schizophrenic faced with the malfunction of his mind, it is deeply and rightly satisfying to be able to relieve it at once and with certainty. This, and not insensitivity to deeper human processes, is the first and sufficient justification of research on psychoactive drugs. Mental symptoms are self-aggravating; doctor or psychiatrist should be ready to break all accessible vicious circles, and we would all welcome sure-fire drug therapy for such predominantly psychogenic symptoms as asthma or impotence, which perpetuate themselves if unchecked. If pharmacology could deal radically with schizophrenia, whatever the true genetic, psychic and biochemical priorities in its causation, a load would be lifted off Man.

Drugs have enormously increased our capacity to help the mentally disturbed. They can often lift the burden of depression, especially chronic, unrecognized depression which the patient and the doctor both experience as vague malaise, lassitude, dysphoria and disinterest. Often these are taken for granted—especially in the old—and only recognized for what they are when a tricyclic or an MAO inhibitor lifts the burden. Antipsychotic agents do not make schizophrenics sane, but they can make the difference between social functioning and life-long hospitalization. Even so-called "senile" dementia is now seen as a disease (of acetylcholinergic transmission, whereas depression and schizophrenia appear to be mediated at least in part by disturbance in other neurotransmitters) and potentially open to drug palliation.

Even more striking is the effect on the so-called borderline patient, whose reactions are multifarious but always inappropriate: we are coming to realize that very often he or she is not so much a product of unfortunate early experience as the medical equivalent of a motorist who is driving a "lemon." The capers and the crazy-making behaviors spring from attempts to control a brain which the patient knows to be unreliable through bitter experience. If the right drug can be found, whether a minimal dose of an antipsychotic, an antidepressant, or an unexpected agent such as thyroxin or ritalin, the faulty connection can be reconnected and the patient's behavior transformed (not always, but we cannot always find the right medication). The advance of neurochemistry will widen our choice and hopefully increase the percentage of successes. We know when success has been attained, because the patient begins to fire on all cylinders and can for the first time benefit from counseling.

At the same time there is something in Eissler's warning, the abuse of psychopharmacology apart. He points out that as physical public health and medicine have suppressed diseases without radically reforming the human environment towards healthiness, so the very successes of psychopharmacology could, if we do not educate ourselves, suppress the ill effects of the social environment without expanding the insight to alter it. This we are beginning to derive from the slower, chancier and grittier business of depth psychology and human ethology. A pill to make everyone fatuously content might not destroy all human initiative, but it would divert attention away from the beginnings which post-Freudian and post-Darwinian man has made in the process of insightful self-comprehension. Something similar applies to the patient who can be tranquilized to the point where he stops making the attempt at communication expressed in his symptom or his appeal for help. Pain-killers are to be welcomed in toothache, but they are not a remedy, still less a program of dental hygiene.

This is a biologically critical decision. If when a social or emotional remedy is needed, we switch to a purely technological answer, we cut off the capacity for planned change. Under the influence of palliatives, society could then go on becoming more and more biologically intolerable and emotionally warped until the palliative itself ran out. The simple analogy of noise, tension and the distribution of sleeping pills is a warning—if we rely on the pills alone we shall increase the dose and the noise-level to the point where toxicity or physical injury supervenes. A tranquilized public will not restrain its most paranoid members by the exercise of active resistance until it is too late.

The Doctor's Problem

The answer is simple enough—we need both biochemical and psychosocial knowledge, the second to use and avoid misusing the first. And the problem of the doctor is no different from that of the unhappy patient, or of man in general—he needs to be adult enough both to use his intellect and to comprehend and be able to experience his emotions. Proper teaching designed both to impart good psychotherapeutic methods and to give the student insight into his own mind and motives, could go a long way to kill those defense mechanisms within the medical man which give us the slaphappy administrator of pills, the veterinary behavior therapist, the brain-washer, the God-omnipotent counselor, and generally, the man who acts out at his patient's expense.

When psychiatrists first introduced this type of instruction into the medical course, there were alarmingly many who could not stand the pace and experience the unpleasant emotions necessary for self-knowledge. Those who did and could, emerged as much better doctors, not only in the field of psychiatry.

Like our patients, we need to be shaken into unhappiness to become fully human.

Anxiety In Adults

For nearly two hundred years it has been an important part of our duty as technicians of public health to make people anxious about themselves and their children. The reasons which lead us to do this were and are morally unexceptionable. When one knows better than one's fellow men, there is both satisfaction and obligation in warning them, and these are redoubled when our fellow men actually employ us for that very purpose. I would like to deal here with the nature of the obligation, and with some of the dangers of the accompanying satisfaction.

The public duty of medicine in the late 18th and early 19th centuries was fairly clear. It knew extremely little, but it was learning more. Its best practitioners, men like Heberden and John Hunter, although they lacked discursive Freudian knowledge of the very subtle dialogue which takes place, unspoken, between physician and patient, had a very clear empirical awareness of it. They knew as well as we do that patients seek not only reassurance but also things for which they do not explicitly ask—parental rebuke or permission, magical transformation, punishment and even death. They also realized, from the sanity of their public and private counsel, that doctors being human have exactly the same needs: from the acrimonious public controversy in which they engaged, according to the manner of the times, they were aware that doctors, no less than others, can be extreme, disturbed, fanatic, and indeed mad. And they had no doubt at all—indeed, they would have welcomed the fact in the true 18th century spirit of classicism—that doctors are a part of the society they live in, and share both its achievements and its quirks.

The use of anxiety which these great forebears made in their office and in their writings[1] was overwhelmingly a sane use. Fothergill and Heberden discovered that the paints and pencils given to children contained lead and arsenic, and that when (in Fothergill's words) "the pernicious implements were taken away," cases of unexplained colic recovered. This applied also to cider in lead-glazed jars. If, as was soon to be shown, sewage in water causes cholera and rats in cities spread plague, the community has every duty to be anxious until rational measures have been taken to remove the nuisance. We today may properly wish that our fellow citizens were more rationally anxious about the carcinogenic effects of cigarette smoking and the long-term results of dumping radioactive matter in the sea. In some cases our counsel is probably wrong, though it is the best we can give at the moment. Alerted businessmen in America have been switched off butter onto corn oil margarine, thence to fish oil, and thence to linseed oil, and back to butter, in the interest of their cholesterol metabolism. Their willingness to follow such stop-press advice is a measure of our prestige as scientists. The cigarette example is a contrary instance—of the power of unconscious and other forces to make not only the patient but his adviser (there must be cigarette smokers reading this) anxiety-proof in certain directions.

The danger of anxiety-making is the danger of all counseling. For our profession it has been particularly acute for a number of reasons. In some matters and at some times we really have known better. Patients singly and collectively have had better insight into the nature of transference than have the medical adherents of scientism. They have expected us to be directive, to discharge the functions of our ancestor the magician, to order unpleasant abstinences and observances, to cut them open and remove not only their appendices but their sins, and today, literally, to put a new heart in them. We have been obliged to play a double game. We do in fact and for sound scientific reasons remove a man's organs and replace them, drill holes in his skull, inject crystals into his tissues, permit him to see his skeleton, make him regress to infancy while we adopt the posture of an Ancestor, or cut off his foreskin. The last is an excellent example—we talk about cleanliness and the elimination of penile carcinoma, and we do so with statistical justification. But all the procedures I have listed are archetypal functions of the aboriginal wizard, who enacts in fantasy those of them which his surgical technique does not permit him to enact in fact, and inside every doctor and patient is an aboriginal trying to get out. Lest we find this worrying, let me remind you that pure science and applied engineering have the same duplicity of viewpoint. The Eskimo wizard receives a call, puts on a suit and mask fit for an other-worldly undertaking, makes a trial flight around the globe, and finally flies to the Moon on a ladder of arrows (a lovely name for a multi-stage launch vehicle) in order to bring back medicine from his spirit bride. If he could make a phallic rocket the size of the Washington Monument, or mate with a mother-vehicle in space, he would no doubt do so. As things are, he does these things more economically than we, but with just as great satisfaction, in fantasy.

What I have written so far is a preface to what I have to say about anxiety. It is commonly said that "anxiety" as a clinical condition is an important public health problem at the present time. What is meant by anxiety is a performance-impairing state of physical and mental alarm which is easier to recognize than to define, which is particularly intense in cultures with a high rate of social and customary change, and which, in its digestive, sexual and other manifestations, as well as in free-floating form, may account for some 90 per cent of the work of the urban general practitioner. We no doubt have our own preference (rarely a research-based preference) for the particular features of modern society which are to blame.

Anxiety Predisposed

Now people have always been anxious. The predisposition is built into man. Primitives have a subtle and sophisticated technology of ceremony and observance to allay this tendency, whether it expresses anxieties common to all—death, Oedipal fears, insecurity—or those special to a culture, such as famine. The wars of the Aztecs were directed to obtain prisoners without whose hearts for food the Gods would die and the seasons stop. The Aztecs are an object-lesson in the gross transformation of primitive magic by civilized societies. There are comparable examples in our own time.

The emotional technology of primitives can take ugly forms: the relatively easy-going religion of the Middle Ages did not prevent epidemics of factional war and persecution or the hunting down of supposed witches and heretics. Medicine only became deeply involved in this cycle at the start of the 19th century and among the independent and increasingly rationalist Protestants of northern Europe. People in the 1800's were increasingly accepting the principle of do-it-yourself change. Idols of many kinds were falling, and with them the authority of priests, kings, aristocrats, confessors. Even religion was a do-it-yourself business drawing authority from the reader's colloquy with God and his interpretation of the scriptures. Every man was to be a father-figure to his wife and children, and the middle classes, representing right-thinking society, were to be father-figures to the dirty, spontaneous and dangerous working classes, who had just decapitated King Louis, but *public* fathers were in short supply. The prestige of the conventional professionals was declining, but that of the doctor and the scientist was growing—the doctors and scientists themselves knew it.

From this situation arose an entire medical posture, which characterized the 19th century, that lasted until Freud, and from which our profession has only just begun to extricate itself. It was in fact the state of paternalist medicine in which the doctor used the authority of his profession to work the oracle in favor of his own or his subculture's prejudices and opinions. The foci of anxiety-making were those normal to the human species. An entire generation was terrorized, not over the sinfulness of sexuality, which is a fully traditional theme, but over its status as a danger to public health. I don't want to go over these excesses in detail—I have documented them elsewhere,[2] in the matter of masturbational insanity, an entirely iatrogenic disease, which led to the castration of a few mental patients and the terrorization of innumerable parents and children; or in the matter of William Acton's rebuke to a patient who thought he could go unscathed in the face of his indulgence in marital intercourse three times within one week. The record of the abuse of medical authority makes ill reading, but there is no point, for its own sake, in mocking the nonsenses of our ancestors. The only object of such a study is to recognize the syndrome and acquire insight into our own more current nonsenses.

A large part of clinical medicine, though it is directive, and almost the whole of the new and growing field of non-directive counseling, is concerned with removing anxieties in our patients—anxieties generated by their past experience, by society, by events, by other physicians. This is an educative function. It depends partly upon giving the facts where we know them, or where we do not, the best that we can. The psychotherapeutic ritual adapted to our society itself depends largely on explanation, because in a discursive culture we need explanation to permit ourselves to feel. Partly also it depends on the attempt to achieve self-acceptance. This too is public health education—whether conducted through books and lectures or through the clinical interview. The paternalist concept of instruction handed down is dead, so far as the growth of modern medicine is concerned. It should be dead in practice. Counseling in modern terms—and the M.O.H. is as much a counselor as the psychiatrist—includes the awareness of such phenomena as reaction-formation and acting-out in application to the counselor as well as to the patient. This awareness is the difference between real counseling, real education, and anxiety-making, which is an exploitation by the doctor of the counseling situation to enable him to experience power or achieve satisfaction. I do not believe that it is difficult to draw the line. That ability depends on the very complex behavioral attribute known as *judgment*, the attribute which John Hunter possessed and William Acton (who was a most humane and upright man) lacked. The danger of bad judgment is perpetual. It can afflict the militant liberal as well as the militant moralist. It is no better for our judgment to be obsessed for personal reasons with the desirability of permissiveness than to be obsessed with the moral ills of self-abuse. Both departures from judgment are unconscious faces of the same currency, and that currency is unconscious anxiety in the doctor himself.

If you share that judgment you will be able to identify some exemplary nonsenses current today. Let me select two counseling instances where we have the choice between genuine counsel and anxiety-making. Oral contraceptives are unsuitable for a certain number of patients and possibly dangerous to a very few. There are great practical and psychological advantages in their use by many, but for others they have psychological drawbacks based on unconscious attitudes to risk, pregnancy and childbirth. They have been more widely and critically tested than any other medicament, but they are by nature active over a long fraction of the taker's endocrine lifespan. It is clearly necessary to assess their likely or observed side effects, and adverse findings should receive due weight. At the same time, nobody could possibly assert that had deep-seated medical anxieties not been aroused by the risk of a safe and continuous control over pregnancy, doctors would have been as cagey as they have been. Do cornflakes or toothpaste predispose to thrombosis? If they do, it has occurred to nobody to ask in the same terms. When we read a paper describing the carcinogenic effects of frying oil, we may look to see if the author is employed by an oil manufacturer, but we do not need to try to guess his religious affiliation from his name. The reason that the Pill inspires our professional caution is not only that it involves the manipulation of little-known endocrines, though this is true. Were reproduction not involved, we would swallow it, and urge others to do so. The real Klansman concealed in this woodpile is our professional awareness that freedom of choice may be being increased. Floodgates are being opened by the thin ends of wedges. This makes us anxious, if we are anxious doctors, and we are confronted by the temptation to frighten others in sympathy. In such a context the only people more unscrupulous than the devout are the frightened, and often they are the same people.

Drug Addiction

The other salient example is that of drug addiction. It is a harder test of our judgment, because there is here a real evil—as often, in cases where we have to choose between judgment and anxiety-making—and consequently the damage we may do if our judgment is inadequate may be considerable. Nobody can be complacent that young men and women are becoming commonly addicted to heroin. We are complacent if our colleagues and national leaders are addicted to alcohol. At the same time, there is in the tone of many official and medical pronouncements so patent an expression of the emotional pleasures of denunciation, so evident an acting-out of the conflict of generations which figured in the literature of masturbational insanity, that we need to take ourselves in hand. There are two courses open: society can react to the problems raised by addictives on one hand and by psychedelics on the other (anxiety-makers aim first to confuse them) by investigation, education and judicious control; or it can react in the spirit of the pussyfoot demanding prohibition. The pussyfoot has no true concern for the alcoholic, for society, or for alcohol as a psychosocial problem. His prime motive is the emotional satisfaction derived from the act of denunciation, however humane the secondary intent. If we tackle the drug problem when we ourselves are intoxicated by distaste for the young (visualized as hippies), fear of substances which release irrationality because we fear our own, and general paternalism, we shall create damage as great to our own society as Prohibition caused to America of the 1920's. This is two-way traffic. The unreason of the addict is plain enough to us, but if our unreason is plain to the younger generation they will defy us on principle and ignore even important and salutary warnings. If we pretend that marijuana "leads to hard drugs" without qualification, we shall bring that effect to pass. (And of course, in America, for fear of sounding like a pussyfoot, we shall ignore alcohol, which is bulkwise if not individually our most deleterious drug of abuse, and treat it as a normal index of sociality largely because our laws are made not by acid-heads but by drinkers, and because some of us use it ourselves.) This does not mean that in the interests of liberty we should abolish drug laws and give lysergic acid to babies and borderline psychotics. It means simply that between the fathead and the acid-head there is a golden mean of unexcited medical judgment, and that this should be the basis of our legislation and health education. I wish I thought we would get it.

Lest you mistake my intention in citing these two examples, let me take a different one. Liberal enthusiasms can themselves create as much anxiety as repressive enthusiasms. If our own reaction to our unconscious problems is to demand the maximum of self-expression, we can foster anxiety in our less-driven patients. Sexual counseling as we know it originated in the need to neutralize older nonsenses by convincing people that they were able, and indeed programmed, to enjoy normal sexuality without guilt. But such is the human appetite for anxiety that reiteration of this salutary principle, in America at least, is producing a fair number of people who are anxious for fear that they are not matching up in frequency, intensity or variety of satisfaction to an arbitrary norm. And then there is child-rearing. The mother who in Victorian times had convinced herself that infantile masturbation would corrupt her child may now convince herself that a brief maternal absence in the hospital will make the child neurotic.

We cannot obviously abolish anxious people. We need to think seriously about their existence whenever we undertake—for example—a campaign of education for early detection of cancer. Carcinophobia is itself an appalling disease, but it is worth a calculated risk if we can help a majority. That is not what I mean by anxiety-making. What has to be avoided in counseling and in public health education is the pronouncement, however factually sound, which ministers in some way to our own anxieties as doctors, or which ministers without our being fully aware of the fact to the paternal and shamanic parts of the medical relationship (these, let me repeat, are real parts, and essential to the relationship, however science-based: they are dangerous only when we fail to recognize them or deny their existence out of excessive confidence in our status as detached scientists). Large numbers of patients with cardiovascular disease are rendered impotent annually for lack of a clear statement that sexual activity can and should be resumed. They may not ask—the burden of positive reassurance rests on us.

So far I have mentioned only iatrogenic anxiety, and in doing so I have really been distinguishing "anxiety" as an endemic psychiatric problem, an unproductive or a disadaptive state of mind, from rational apprehension. It is quite easy to create anxiety about the existence of anxiety in our culture, putting it down to whatever feature of the culture we ourselves find unacceptable. Pressures of urban living are a fairly common candidate. In 1857 John Hawkes, assistant medical officer of Wilts County Asylum, wrote:

> I doubt if ever the history of the world...could show a larger amount of insanity than that of the present day...It seems as if the world was moving at an advanced rate of speed proportionate to its approaching end...a higher pressure is engendered on the minds of men.

Notice the eschatological overtone. We know a little about the origins of individual anxiety in upbringing and childhood experience, and this psychoanalytic insight is clinically useful. But we have no social psychiatry to match, and the feedback between society and family, society and the person, is clearly gross.

From the broader public health point of view we need a great deal more knowledge. The situations producing stress diseases in monkeys are highly specific; it is not enough to denounce features of society which appear on general grounds to be a source of stresses. It is difficult to find an index of anxiety—to admit or show oneself anxious may be the convention of one culture in expressing stress, where a different culture or another person describes the experience as physical illness. Mental disorder may or may not be a proper index of what we are trying to measure. Leighton[3] compared the incidence of overt mental illness in urban and rural Yoruba and Americans—the chief correlation is with weakness or rapid change in social organization. Rawnsley[4] attempted to unravel and compare the psychiatric and psychosomatic contributions to medical consultations in different regions of England, and to explain, for example, the very high incidence of psychiatric illness in some Welsh mining valleys. There are too many conclusions possible here for us to jump to any of them. Apart from general social influences, it is worth looking for specific stresses which predispose to specific symptoms or diseases—these may be quite circumscribed, like the conditions which produce ulcers in "executive" monkeys. Stress at least is physiologically measurable, if we care to define our terms. "Anxiety" and "anxiety states" are far more general names for the sense of something amiss, where even subjective assessment is hazardous, and where the willingness to admit to the experience may be an actual alternative to physical disease, and as such, of service to the patient.

There remains the truth that general tranquilization is not our function, any more than the insightless exploitation of human fears. It is unnecessary to make people anxious, it is sometimes necessary to permit them to experience and admit anxiety, it is sometimes necessary to foster rational apprehension—of the kind which leads to rational action—over such matters as preventable damage to the environment, overpopulation, misuse of drugs, and psychiatrically insightless social or personal behavior. On the basis that fear is discharged by rational action, we shall be right if we control our own private anxieties and counsel from a just combination of thinking and feeling. We shall be wrong, even if we are nominally right, where our counseling is judgmental or subserves private ends.

Thinking and Feeling

I believe that the real psychiatric and philosophical problem of modern societies lies in adjusting the balance between thinking and feeling. This is especially true of medicine, which tries as no other specialty to be both rational and insightful. Primitives have their technologies of dealing with the emotions, but can do little about the environment. Industrial man has acquired nearly unlimited powers of dealing with the environment, but the necessary effort of practical abstraction has caused him to lose touch with the overt expression of feelings, so that when emotional motives appear in his medicine, his engineering and his town-planning they do so unacknowledged. The problem of cybernetic man, with which psychoanalysis and ethology have made some kind of start, is that of applying reason to understand our emotions without the necessity of denying them. This ought not to be impossible, and we have made a beginning. That beginning is the real basis of the change in the posture of medicine.

Perhaps I might appropriately end with some words which I borrow from a report by Rosemary Firth, of the London Institute of Education, which sums up my argument regarding health education. She writes:

"The medical profession in this country, as elsewhere, is continually expressing its public anxiety about the choices open to people in evading or treating illness. But they are not willing..." [may I interpolate, some in the past have not been willing]..."to provide a real opportunity for the public to make 'free' choices; they wish to 'force' the choices according to the medical world's idea of a patient-doctor relationship...All this adds up to the simple conclusion that health education to be effective implies giving the public information, and allowing them to discuss and evaluate their own problems of health and disease. Health education at the level of manipulation of behavior by the onesided presentation of facts designed to persuade people out of fear or cowardice to act in certain ways—e.g. refrain from sexual promiscuity or smoking or drinking—is bound to be ineffective because inefficient in the modern world."[5]

Possibly Dr. Firth should change her physician, for this is a conclusion with which I feel most public health educators will now agree. But it does no harm to point the moral. Where our own anxieties are concerned, mine as well as yours, there is a normative force in the consensus of balanced opinion.

References
1. Fothergill, J. Collected Works. London, John Walker, 1781.
2. Comfort, A. The Anxiety Makers. London, Nelson, 1967.
3. Leighton, A.H. *In* Platt, R. and Parkes, A.S.: Social and genetic influences on Life and Death. Edinburgh and London, Oliver & Boyd, 1967.
4. Rawnsley, K. *Ibid.*, 1967.
5. Firth, R. Communication circulatd in typescript, 1968.

"Sex and Violence" in Psychiatry
(Three talks to psychiatric residents)

You may be relieved or disappointed to hear that very little of what I am going to say in these three talks is going to be of much help to you in dealing with multiple-choice examinations. In England, before letting psychiatrists loose on the public, we make them write essays to ensure that they are literate. You may well be relieved rather than disappointed that nothing of the kind will be expected of you. The subject I was originally asked to talk about was "overdetermination"— meaning the fact that the same symbolisms and behaviors may mean different things to different patients, and usually mean or derive their power from more than one of these things. I chose to use "sex and violence"—or more correctly the problem of the meaning of what are traditionally called "sadomasochistic" behaviors—partly because I thought a prurient title would ensure that residents would turn up regardless of the inutility of the course for Brownie points, and partly because I wanted a concrete example of what overdetermination means from an area in which I had collected some data. One of the reasons for collecting data, as you will find, is to have a field of concrete observation from which you can draw lecture examples.

I have divided this brief course into three areas—roughly "fantasy and literature", "play and drama", and "idiosyncrasy and magic"—revolving in each case around the same group of perplexing behaviors, the interaction of sexuality and aggression. The fact that I am leaving out more conventional explanations of that group of behaviors is simply that my colleagues have dealt with them already. You can add them to your list of overdeterminants.

If you want a different and more definite example of overdetermination, consider the salmon-fly. It is a concoction of feathers and tinfoil offered to a salmon at a time when that animal is not feeding, so it is not mistaken for food. It has been empirically devised so that, although it does not resemble anything a salmon has ever seen before, it excites a range of fishy responses, including (probably) curiosity, aggression, desire and—for all we know, not being salmon—sexual attraction sufficiently strong to make the salmon attack, or at least investigate it.

A sexual object—whether person, fetish or behavior-pattern—is a very similar stimulus. There are some traits, connected with reminiscence, texture, and expected physical sensation, which make such an object attractive either generally or to a subgroup of people. There are others which may be biologically programmed—a limited number of hooks on which sexual cathexis may be hung, just as there are a limited number of physical manipulations effective in producing or enhancing orgasm. Some people go heavily for one of these aspects, and we may be able to make Freudian sense of the reasons in experience which may make them do so.

But however large such a determinant, the others are there too. Straight heterosexual preferences have large time-and-culture determinants. Fetishes, though by definition idiosyncratic and very rigid in that individuals who show them do not switch them around, are limited in number and rather highly canalized: the individual who gets his satisfaction from climbing into a bath of cooked spaghetti or thinking about safety pins is rare. There is, in other words, a repertoire of feathers from which, once simple selection of an opposite-sex partner is overridden, a suitable fly can be tied. Prostitutes and pornographers are empirical experts in the manipulation of these "polymorphous-perverse" elements, and most of us respond larvally to some of them when attached to, rather than divorced from, another eligible human being.

A good example of a potent overdetermined structure with which we are all familiar, personally or by proxy, is the erect penis. A simple Martian might expect it to be exciting to females and boring, by familiarity, to males. Experience and Freud show us that this is not so. It may be interesting to females at appropriate moments and attached to the right person, but far more generally it is boring to females and exciting, or a subject of solicitous anxiety, to males. In phylogeny, and in humans, it is a dominance signal, which explains the anxieties of male patients about its size and predictability. It is a reassurance against castration—for some, whose own is insufficient, it may be a fetish necessary to physical desire. This is true of some (but not by any means all) predominantly homosexual males. It may, in the presence of great insecurity, be replaceable by surrogates—show me a "gun lobby" nut, and I will show you a sexually apprehensive male. In other words, function, selfestimate, sociobiological restes and Freudian psychodynamics all revolve around it—making man, incidentally, unique in attaching so much importance to a primary, and so little importance to secondary, sex characteristics. Nobody writes about beard envy.

These examples show what we mean by overdetermination. Now let us begin.

The Warrior and the Suffragette
Notes of the science fiction of John Norman

There are some fantasies, or climates of fantasy, which are pervasive. Like air pollution or an ethnic dietary preference, they affect the generality. One of these is the nexus of feelings, largely irrational, which affect the notions we have of, and the relations we fantasy between, Manhood and Womanhood. On paper these may look rarefied. In fact, they leak into the practice of medicine from all sides. Quite apart from usual sexual dysfunctions, the seas of feminism, intersexual hostility, new attitudes, loud propaganda, traditional male cowboyism and changing socioeconomic reality break over patients, disturbing their fantasy-based marital fortresses, bedeviling their fantasy-based self-images, giving them additional coupons for hypertension, ulcers and "diazepam deficiency" and, incidentally, wasting a lot of your office time.

They also explode intermittently in society. Your female patients will be quite reasonably concerned about rape. Others will present with recurrent unexplained injuries—if you are alert to battered babies, you will recognize them as victims of domestic violence which they will often inexplicably try to prevent you from detecting. You will notice these cases more often if you stop believing that illiterates and the impoverished beat their wives, while graduates and the prosperous do not.

Much violence in our society represents very natural frustration and hatred. On one hand is the folk fantasy that anyone can succeed and get his share of the goodies in our free and competitive society: those who can't and don't may react by practical social militancy, or by mere envy, or by comprehensible but ill-directed anger (for those whose fault is in themselves rather than in their stars, usually the last). A common motive of rape is envy with low self-esteem rather than mere Freudian aggression or mother-figure bashing: in this regard it resembles bank robbery or automobile theft. The cultural fantasy has reduced women to the status of desirable, prestige-conferring objects, and intercourse, like wealth, to a measure of success. For the man who can get neither, or believes he can get neither, but is surrounded by those who have both, woman is a provocation and a taunt—not by being provocative or seductive, as some retarded judges think, but simply by being there.

If a fantasy can give a man ulcers or make the streets unsafe for our inoffensive wives and sisters, fantasies are clearly part of the web of public health, as significant as sewer lines and bovine tubercle in milk. Like so many other nonconcrete determinants of health and disease, doctors cannot do a great deal about them: one cannot remove or modify them by disinfection or even legislation, but one can study them wherever possible—in ourselves as well as in our society.

There are various ways of doing this. Introspection is one—but it is difficult to see into one's own ears. If we engage in much counseling, we shall actually hear fantasies expressed. If we use our eyes in watching television and movies and in inspecting the contents of bookshops, we can learn about the anthropology of our own culture—and here it is not so much art and literature but bad B movies and pop magazines which tell us most. We can learn explicit psychology from Tolstoy or Shakespeare or Goethe, but we can learn about popular fantasy from Tarzan, Spiderman, King Kong and *Redbook,* from *Playboy* and the gun collectors' journals, for all of these, at their different levels of achievement, have been sharpened by commercial natural selection to speak for the fantasies of those who patronize them. Human natural history is a field in which observation can begin with what is on the waiting room table.

I take the example of sexuality and aggression because it is socially disquieting, and because it crops up, when one gets to the counseling level, in unexpected people and with unexpected frequency. Psychoanalysts and sociobiologists have run themselves ragged over it: neurologists point out that adjacent limbic functions might well be expected to "bleed over" between channels—that both have a common component in desire, arousal, and dominance behavior. That still doesn't explain why fantasies of rape are common in liberated and unmasochistic women who regard male domination as an anachronistic insult and display high self-esteem and confidence. Not all of these patients can have overheard parental copulation and mistaken it for violence; what is going on?

A number of psychoanalysts, notably Robert Stoller,[1,2] have been preoccupied with this problem, and have written in Jeremiac terms about the covert, as well as the overt, violence implicit in pornography—with the conclusion that all sexual love requires a small component of hate to act, as it were, in the role of detonator. It is not clear whether this is seen as a general, "sociobiological" truism or simply a criticism of contemporary American gender fantasies. "Love," in the sense in which we use it of lifelong emotional commitment based on sexual attraction, is ethnographically rather a rare human experience. We evolved in a context where women have been more often valued for their fertility or their digging ability than as sex objects, and we might be paying the penalty for upgrading the concept of male-female association to a civilized level.

I want to pursue this example as an object lesson in the medico-psychiatric study of "human natural history": first, because I myself was profoundly surprised in researching a counseling book by the widespread incidence of pseudoaggressive fantasy in non-dysfunctional people; second, because it has some clinical interest; and third, because it indicates how the nonpsychiatric human naturalist can conduct observation on his culture without having to carry out interviews. After going through this example, you will have no difficulty at all in thinking of other fantasy-structures of clinical and social importance where the same approach is feasible. The fantasy of Medicine itself might be a still more interesting exercise. The method begins, where depth interviewing is impracticable, by looking at popular literature.

Storytelling is one of the most important of human cultural mechanisms. Through it we impart tradition and the "set" of a culture—in preliterate orders we can learn most of how it feels to grow up within them by learning their stories. The physician, who needs every source of information, should look at such evidence. How far we could learn what modern America is like by reading its storytelling literature, as against its "serious" writers, is another matter. Our fiction, in its preoccupation with violence, is certainly self-revelatory, and it certainly transmits cultural attitudes. It also, however, serves the other important function of storytelling, the expression of fantasy—the depiction not of what the culture expresses but of what it suppresses.

While gnomic storytelling is a way of transmitting mores, the literature of fantasy is amoral. Through it impoverished cultures share the exploits of fabulously rich kings, and helpless cultures the omnipotence of wizards and heroes. The greatest popular literature oscillates between the real and wish, between mores and the hidden fantasy. Perhaps our finest example is in the Arabian Nights, which combine sharp insight into 16th century Arabian cultures with marvellous adventure, folk tales with literary satire, Islamic devotion with total opportunism, and overall an aura of psychosexual excitement which was less evident to the original hearers of the tales than to our culture, where they carry the association of exoticism and its attendant permissions.

Our equivalent is hokum, and for the purpose of this study the form of hokum which we can most creatively examine is science fiction.

Some of this, of course, is not hokum at all, but now that we have jet planes the exotic is of necessity either historical or extraterrestrial in site. Like the folk tale, science fiction serves both normative and anomic needs. On one hand it can be a fictional science hypothesis which explores possible technology, often in a spirit of warning (Faust was a science fiction hero), or the social comment implicit in Utopias and Dystopias. On the other, it has access to the mainstay of all hokum, the far country where sexual fantasy becomes fact, the role which Turkey played to the readers of 18th century romances, or ancient Rome to the readers of *Quo Vadis?*

I have argued elsewhere[3] that literature does not degenerate into hokum—often it is the backbone of hokum, of that which is psychosymbolically exciting, which provides the stimulus of literature. And of all topics which make hokum work, it is the uneasy association between sexuality and violence or suffering, the Perils of Pauline, the Misfortunes of Virtue, which seems to carry the highest audience appeal. The perils and misfortunes which bring women (in the mythology of hokum) to arousal may be magical or romantic, urbane like Snow White or frankly sadistic as in the *Story of 'O'*. With the demythologizing of sexuality, sex and violence are now becoming just that—the violence was always respectable, however, and most of the censure is directed at the fact that some sexual reference is now explicit, and the heroine gets laid as well as tortured. Provided it does not get close enough to actuality to be disturbing, and even now, when it does, there is nothing like sadomasochism to make a story go.

Many writers of science fiction in its hokum, Arabian Nights or comic book mode dilute this theme with gentler or more disguised fantasy material. At least one of them tackles it head on and with a good deal of insight into the psychosymbolism of his genre, borrowing verisimilitude from extensive reading on ancient naval tactics, linguistics, cryptography—even biology, although he has some six-legged mammals which would not stand up (in more ways than one). His heroes, like Sinbad, even ride on tarns—giant eagles—the descendants of the roc and the simurgh.

John Norman, an excellent storyteller and a university lecturer, has created an anti-planet ("Gor") devoted to the enactment of sexual fantasy. Its male inhabitants—confined by a wise theocracy of insect priest kings to the military level of Vikings by the prohibition of any weapon more lethal than a bow—are free to devote their energies to typical masculine pursuits: fighting and the enslavement of women. Gorean women fall into three categories—slavegirls, who suffer the entire erotic repertoire of the comic books, but become immensely responsive as a result: Panther Girls—Amazons who enslave men, play the warrior role, and despise slave women: and Free Companions (wives, in Earthly parlance) who go veiled, cultivate jealousy, knock their female slaves about with even greater enthusiasm than warriors, and are, with the exception of a few spirited princesses, frigid and rather obnoxious people. Throughout a round dozen of stories, the recurrent theme is the inhibited daughter of Earth, fortunate enough to be abducted by Goreans, who is enslaved, subjected to training similar in detail but more robust in conception to that undergone at Roissy by the amoeboid "O", compelled into sexual response, and who discovers her true femininity in abandoning intellectual and social competition with men and embracing a delicious servitude to a succession of warriors (Motherhood is not part of the erotic feminine experience—Gorean slavegirls are kept on a contraceptive potion and permanently nubile, gerontology being a technology to which the priest kings have no objection).

An anti-world is of course a site for the enactment not of the real but of the hidden and the unperformed. Although Mr. Norman philosophizes about the sexually emancipating effects of female submission almost as much as Paulhan, he is obviously not giving a prescription for society.

Quite a lot of the cover story is well done, though the stigmata of hokum are present and by the 13th volume the ideas flag badly: the plotting is careless and a pretext, as in the charades of lovers, for the psychosexual kicks. The novels, moreover, fall off individually with the iteration of the theme of erotic subjection—the tarns, which figure in the first novel, are a splendid and archetypal fantasy which enable us to tolerate the musclebound condottiere who ride on them: hokum is no bar to good fictional ideas, as Flaubert showed in *Salammbô*. Embarrassing overwriting is also a convention of much science fiction, where it avoids the whimsy of Tolkien or the archness of C.S. Lewis, and Norman pulls out all the stops:

"In the course of the savage discipline inflicted on me" [writes a Norman heroine of a gang-rape] "I had...sensed the ancient primate complementarity of male and female....I a female was simply subordinate to the male. I...experienced an incredible sense of freedom, of liberation, not the freedom of convention but the freedom of nature, not the freedom to be what I was not, which had been prescribed to me, but the freedom rather to be what I was...the freedom of a rock to fall, of a flower to bloom."

And later: "You want to be conquered and enslaved, don't you, you slut?" he said.

"Yes" I said, "I am a woman."

(*Slavegirl of Gor*, 1977)

As for the Panther Girls, who react quite reasonably to this philosophy by playing macho, they only attain Gorean femininity when subdued, enslaved, and enabled thereby to achieve total orgasm, which is possible only when they accept the status of joyful chattels, and only with a male who they know to be capable of unpredictable tenderness and unpredictable brutality by turns—in Gorean terms a natural male. Free Companions, moreover, when preorgasmic, respond to the same treatment and re-enlist as slavegirls to realize their rejected femininity.

What are we to make of this stuff, and why do humans chronically read it? Feminists would be inclined to see the entire fantasy as an indiscreetly explicit expression of the true cultural attitude of men towards women—hostility masquerading as sentiment. History provides them with a great deal of ammunition. Barroom biology, sophisticated or unsophisticated, while admitting that we have outgrown that sort of thing now, suggests that aggression in the male and submission in the female were at some time adaptive, and that we have retained the wiring—whence the response. Norman is himself long on this type of biology—whereas Justine was the victim of simple cruelty for kicks, in the name of 18th century amoralism, his mistreated heroines are recovering their primate heritage. The trouble with this is that the primate heritage, along with the cartoon figure of the "cave man" who knocks his partner down with a club, are themselves fantasy-formations with absolutely no basis in observed behavior, either of primates or of primitive man, for hokum is cerebral and the product of cultures which are out of touch with the physical—this in itself explains part of our fascination with violence, for although we have plenty of that, it is mediated by weapons which limit the physical expression of aggression to pulling triggers or even to signing papers.

We get a truer picture of the role of aggression, both hostile and appetent, in physical societies by reading the Sagas. Viking life was often nasty, brutish and brief, but its fantasies transcend rather than cultivate those qualities. Joy of battle is an unpopular emotion in our culture, and rightly, in a world of atomic bombs, but in any case it is the enjoyment of violence as self-testing, not as a cerebral excuse for sexual kicks.

One could of course summarily dismiss the planet Gor as the inner world of insecure males, for whom women prove one too many, subdued by mothers, sisters and sexual partners, and fantasizing rather than meditating an order in which they would recover their virility by reprisals, rather like the hero of Fellini's "8½" who appears as ringmaster to make his demanding mistresses jump through hoops—the male chauvinism of the uncocksure. We must all be not a little disturbed by the fantasy, in view of the increase in hostile behaviors towards women by male inadequates, and the tendency of police and other authorities to see domestic violence—the commonest cause of physical injury to women—as humorous and probably erotic, rather than as terrifying and brutal.

In point of fact, however, the efficacy of Norman's legend is more complicated and more confusing, and it poses questions in human ethology which remain with the reader, for the fantasy which it contains, so far from being confined to inadequate men, is also one of the commonest reported by adequate women: these adventures and The Story of 'O' are among the works which women as well as men report as sexually stimulating. They have even been recommended in counseling works as a source of increased fantasy-capacity for those who fantasize with difficulty or require fictional permission to entertain their erotic fantasies. Modern women, who rightly revolt against a long factual history and a present continuance of brutality against their sex by men, very naturally regard this component of fantasy in both sexes as abominable. Nonsense written in the past about feminine masochism seems to support the reasonableness of their attitude. Unfortunately the fantasies exist, as most counselors are aware, and if we are to prevent their intrusion onto Earth and into actual social behaviors, we need to look at their puzzling ethology. The game of gladiators and slavegirls is a constant and archaic human favorite—it is arousing as play and disgusting as a social style. It is not commonly realized how many of our cultural problems, not only sexual but political, economic and intrapersonal, arise from the treatment of structures appropriate to play as though they were teleonomic and appropriate to real or earnest activities. Therefore if we are to get control of this one, we need to understand it; a difficult task, because it is highly overdetermined, involving a deepseated confusion between appetency and aggression and between sex and violence.

Large tracts of human behavior, sexual and social, do in fact dramatize aspects of the ambivalence of the sexes toward each other. It is the interface between our dominance-based and communication-based primate heritages, between baboonery and chimpanism, if one may coin simpler names for them than "agonic" and "hedonic"—which seems to give us the most trouble in this regard. Sexual aggression, not necessarily involving hostility, and sexual submission, not necessarily involving masochism, do have a superficial look of archaic programming—socialization has made them irrelevant not only in civilized but in practically all human societies, the civilized finding them the most troublesome. But they have become fossilized in the range of

human releaser mechanisms by the fact that our psychosexual development is built from scraps of phylogeny—the father-son dominance
anxiety, for example, which we have displaced into infancy and used,
it appears, as a mechanism in individuation.

It takes only a trifling phylogenetic push to "load" a train of psychosymbolism and to pattern a whole sequence of cultural consequences,
themselves overdetermined and maintained by quite other forces, rather
as a tilt or an irregularity in the foundations can pattern the stresses in a
building. The pattern of ambivalence between men and women, expressed as male uneasiness over the magical threat posed by Woman, is a
Freudian tilt of this kind—a confusion between the signal mechanisms
connected with sexuality and those connected with hostility is an ethological tilt in the same direction, unrelated but contributory.

In fact it is this ethological ambivalence, the double-take between
arousal, aggression, hostility, responsiveness and submission which
may well provide the historically original tilt upon which subsequent
psychoanalytic structures stand. To children, enthusiastic sexual intercourse notoriously looks like assault. The theory which connects adult
confusion between sex and violence, aggression and appetency ("sadomasochism"), with the primal scene seems to be on roughly the right
ethological lines.

Different societies have dealt differently with the awareness of this
double-take. The more likeable have stylized it or translated it into
play, the most effective displacement activity available to humans. We
see this in the widespread use of "marriage by capture," which probably had origins in the proprietary attitude of kin to their womenfolk,
but which serves when ritualized to recognize a deepseated violation-
anxiety, turn it into playful or stylized dramatization and thereby into
arousal by the technique now known to therapists as "flooding." Not
uncommonly these are societies, like Burkhardt's Wahabi,[4] where the
status of women is high and the charade of rape is chiefly erotic horseplay. Our culture limits this ritual to the lifting of the bride over the
threshold (the fact of being lifted bodily is itself an arousing reminiscence—one of the greatest erotic scenes in cinema was where Rhett
Butler carried Scarlett O'Hara upstairs). The only extant anthropological example of Gorean goings-on appears to be the capture ceremony
of the Pokot.[5] In this, women are indeed captured and imprisoned and
have intercourse forced on them; but the performance is ritualized,
and the rapees are volunteers. Britain formerly had a ceremony (Hock-
Tide) where on successive days men captured women and women
captured men, "binding one another and attempting, God forbid,
things even worse and more immodest, holding out that they collect

money for the Church, but getting themselves by the pretense only damnation."*[6] "Binding Tuesday" or Hock-Day was abolished at the Reformation—its actual anthropology is unknown, but it was clearly an occasion for horseplay which addressed the fear of violation through a tolerated suspension of ordinary decencies—those whose fears were real probably stayed indoors, as soberer Hindus do at Holi. Moreover, each sex took a turn, and the women were by tradition the more violent.

More obnoxious societies have acted out gladiators and slavegirls in deadly earnest. Very inhibited societies have bypassed the problem by displacing anxiety onto sex itself, by making it a guilty and a hostile activity, pleasureless for both sexes. The image popular with barroom biology of the "primitive" society as involving brutality to women as a natural or adaptive feature is without any historical basis in anthropology. Comic book societies are as a rule a rare and late development of decadent complex rather than robust and physical styles. When the status of women is low in simple societies they are seen far more as real estate or beasts of burden than as objects for rape. The institution of slavery has been overwhelmingly political and economic in its motives, but in societies afflicted with decay-phase ennui it has at the same time provided women who could be used for fantasy-enactment without recourse—Roman, Ottoman societies and the Old South were cases in point. These societies once provided a fantasy-context in report, like the planet Gor, for the hokum which excited respectable people in Victorian and 18th century England, where Roman and Turkish scenarios took the place of frank science fiction.

One can see the dangerous potential of the material which fantasies of rape and aggression contain. The person to whom they are least disturbing is the sex counselor—not because he underrates the ability of psychopathic characters to enact them in fact, but because he recognizes where they properly belong and is in the business of ensuring that they get put back there.

For a start, sexually oriented enactments of submission and domination, so far from being a "primate heritage" of the female, are just about equally distributed in both sexes, and occur in playful and unhostile people (who enjoy them) as well as in hostile, sadistic or maso-

---

*"Uno certo die heu usitato hoc solempni festo Paschi transacto mulieres homines, alioque die homines mulieres ligare ac cetera media utinam non inhonesta vel deteriora facere moliantur et exercere, lucrum Ecclesiae fingentes sed dampnum animae sub fucato colore lucrantes..."[6]

chistic people (who view them with excitement and anxiety and are hung up on them). Most of them, when enacted, have little or nothing to do with hostility and a great deal to do with muscular eroticism: they are highly overdetermined behaviors—hostile people will use them to express hostility, and guilty people, guilt, but even so they remain within the boundaries of our most important and underrated human behavior, namely *play*.

The function of human play includes the constructive resolution of fantasy. Sexuality is one of its most important theaters—it is the adult equivalent of childhood play.

The small child who experiences jealous hostility to a supplanting brother or sister which he may not express has a number of inner resources in dealing with it. He may partially process his unbiddable emotions in dreams. He may express them to himself in fantasies—often of a bloodthirsty sort, which alarm adults when expressed. In play, however, the intrusion of reality disciplines them. He plays at "Bang, you're dead"—but nobody is dead in fact; the tension is translated into motor activity, and he gains both reinforcement and a certain reassurance both as to the worthiness of hostile feelings so transmuted and as to their harmlessness to others. In adults fantasy is an equally worthy resource precisely because it is uncensored and not a scenario for earnest, but for play. Its enactment, however alarming it sounds when the fantasy is verbalized, is moderated at once when translated into sexual play by the physical presence of the partner as playmate, by the restraint implicit in naming a behavior playful, by the need for orgasm and pleasure, and by the genuine "primate heritage" of sexual resources present in Man, whereby simulated aggressions and submissions, role exchanges, and muscular eroticism increase arousal. Sexual play within these limits turns the fantasies of stable and unanxious people into pleasure and bonding, and enables anxious people to overcome anxieties or achieve permission by a pretense of compelling or being compelled by a partner. Our society, by a combination of literalism and antisexuality, is apt to turn originally unhostile wishes into violence because that is "decent" while orgasm is not.

The trouble with literalism is that we are ashamed of admitting that we are playing—and accordingly, people who find particular situational releasers erotic quite often invent scenarios to make their odd behaviors logical, even in the play context. The individuals who enjoy purely sexual submission or domination may need to create a scenario in which they are punished for an imaginary fault, simply to provide a story line. The storyteller who is developing erotic fantasies has to do the same thing, and since the behaviors which are arousing and collusive in the sexual context would be read as hostile in any other non-play and non-sexual context, the story acquires hostile content simply to justify the behaviors—rather as a patient who was excited by dressing in rubber suits for kicks became a skindiver to provide a realistic cover for a behavior which he could not tolerate without a "realistic" explanation.

This fantasy-complex was in fact one of the main problems we had to address in writing The Joy of Sex. Our aim was to give permissions to behaviors which appeared to be resources, and to do this we had to assess the uses most commonly made of them, on Maslow's rule that it is not behaviors, but their significances, which are to be classified as unhelpful or perverse. We were struck by the extreme commonness of play behaviors, both in fantasy and in enactment, which sounded aggressive or masochistic in description but which were wholly playful, and apparently reinforcing, in practical enactment. The distinction is not always realized by therapists who listen to couch descriptions and do not observe, or at least listen carefully to, what is actually done. Divorced from interpretive overlay, scenarios are devised justifying the understood, or from readings by clients of explanatory psychiatric literature (I have heard a man say that he could never allow himself to experience a submissive form of play, because he identified himself in psychiatric literature as a "dominant male"). Compared with all except the anxieties which focus around bisexual response this seemed to us the least understood and least ventilated area of sexual fantasy in our culture. What we learned from examining it was, primarily, the fact that anxieties become pleasures when physically transmuted into play in all but a recognizably preoccupied minority, whose sexual hostility towards self or others is expressed elsewhere—in being down-putters or putdown, in accident-proneness and the like. "Sado-masochism" as a description of this highly overdetermined set of releasers seemed an inappropriately loaded term.

As to the "primate heritage," it is there all right, but not in the form of a battle of the sexes: even if no basic hostilities were present, the scenario would sound hostile, even if the enactment were playful and tender. It is therefore not so odd that normal men and women are aroused by fantasizing active and passive rape, whereas actual rape so far from being arousing is terrifying, humiliating and wholly unerotic.

That, of course, does not remove all anxieties about fantasy literature. We should not take it at its face value, and anyone who recognizes from counseling practice the difference between sexual fantasy on the couch and sexual play on the hoof has the task of giving permission to the first and then encouraging its translation into the second. In spite of the risks which Mr. Norman runs by philosophizing and protesting too much (an embryo Nazi or psychopath might be listening and take him seriously), he recognizes that what he writes is a scenario for play, for he has in fact written a book (*Imaginative Sex*, 1974) in which he specifically suggests the transmutation. Unfortunately, being a child of our time unable to enjoy without explanation, he cannot simply say, "If the fantasy turns you on, try it as a scenario for adult play." Instead he discourses at length on primate heritages, women as the prey of primitive hunters, and much else of like kind. This may serve, like the frog-suit cover, to allay the anxieties of readers and give them permission to be playful, but it is at least as much directed to his own. There is a stamp of uncocksureness in his insistence that male should as a rule subdue female, instead of taking turns, though even his macho heroes are occasionally on the receiving end. As we have said, female pseudoaggression is at least as much a releaser for males as male pseudoaggression is for females. It would not be odd, given the energy with which we have inhibited female response, and the long cultural heritage of keeping one's legs closed which in precontraceptive days had a lot of solid sense on its side, if women more readily got permission to respond through a charade of compulsion, but it does not appear to be the case. The trip laid on men by macho performance anxiety is in some ways heavier than that laid by men on women, and most of them would greet simulated rape by a female with relief; they could lie back and enjoy it.

Accordingly, neither civilized concern nor feminism can get anywhere by suppressing fantasy. The task is to limit the actual expression of hostility in society, and our growing awareness of sexual psychodrama as a resource to bring this about will suffer if our sense of concern is so frightened by the cover-story that we lose the resource. Uncensored, unanxious fantasy combined with creative sexual play are two of the most useful resources we possess in coming to terms with the difficult adjustment of man to woman, woman to man, and both to culturally ingrained anxiety. In this the storyteller has his place, and if hokum is a trigger for unanxious fantasy in either sex it has therapeutic value. After all, the hostile, the sadistic and the disturbed will find fuel for their preoccupations in Shakespeare, the Bible, or the Manhattan phonebook. It is part of the shamanic function of the storyteller to put us back in touch with a genuine "primate heritage"—what we have to be careful about is the keeping of play and earnest, playfulness and acting-out, in separate and labeled compartments.

References

1. Stoller, R.J.: Pornography and perversion. Arch. gen. Psychiat. 22:490-499, 1970.

2. Stoller, R.J.: Sexual excitement. Arch. gen. Psychiat. 33:899-909, 1976.

3. Comfort, A.: Darwin and the Naked Lady. London, Routledge, 1961.

4. Burckhardt, J.L.: Notes on the Bedouins and Wahabys. London, 1830.

5. Conant, F.P.: The external coherence of Pokot ritual and behavior. Phil. Trans. B 251:505-519, 1966.

6. Leland: Collectanea. In Chambers, E.K., The Mediaeval Stage. Oxford, Clarendon Press, 1903.

Sexuality, Play and Earnest

Some of you will be familiar with Jean Genet's play *Le Balcon*. In outline it deals with a brothel whose frequenters have an opportunity to enact their sexual fantasies with the assistance of the staff. A client who is excited by taking the role of a bishop or a general, or who likes his partner to impersonate a nun or a slave-girl, resorts to this establishment as a relief from the prosaic demands of reality. Comes the revolution, however, and the fantasy bishop and the fantasy general find themselves a real bishop, a real general. The brothel has taken over the world: role-playing for kicks becomes full-time. What Genet is suggesting is that there is really no difference between limited role-playing and role-playing in general: fantasy is fantasy, whether we see that or not, and however seriously we take the fantasies we enact.

This is as good a place as any to take up again the problem I raised before concerning the fantasies expressed in popular literature and nourished secretly by all of us, or almost all of us, who have the imagination to fantasize. What Genet has written is a play about play, about the frontiers between play, which allows and discharges fantasy; theatre, which enacts fantasy with a convention of unreality; and "reality" or earnest—which cannot be made a vehicle for aggressive, manipulative and grandiose behaviors if we aim at a reasonably civilized life. Play and fantasy, plays and literature, are safety-valves which wiser people use to avoid treating the world as a theatre. Genet, who had severe problems of his own (he spent many years in jail as a habitual criminal) suggests that it can't be done: a bishop is a bishop for kicks, whether he convinces himself otherwise or not. He would tell you that a physician is a physician for kicks, whether he convinces himself otherwise or not. Well, indeed, our fantasy may be defeating sickness and helping people, in which case good luck to the performance, though we need to be aware of what is going on. Not all human fantasies are as amiable, as we have seen. We are talking here about overdetermination in sexual behaviors, a fairly limited field. Here at least Genet's comments on the theatrical element in sexuality (which, I assure you, is general, and not confined to people who dress up or exhibit unusual preferences) chime well with clinical observation.

Our society is grossly handicapped by literalism. To our aboriginal ancestor all things were magical—stones and animals addressed him, trees were animate, the world in which he lived was that of *L'Enfant et les sortilèges*. There is a duality in his perception—he does not confuse the Great Serpent with real serpents, or the stones of Ayers Rock, which are the bones of magical ancestors, with real bones. These things belong to the Dream Time, those to daily life. He would never, like certain Fundamentalist Christians, set out in search of Noah's Ark.

Literalism is the cultural price we pay for our greatest discovery, namely *science*. So long as we believe that devils cause smallpox, then whatever the diabolic fauna of our own heads we shall fail to cure it. The schoolmen were convulsed for centuries over a concept of matter which would enable bread literally to become flesh. The literalism of great religions, which has brought them from the sphere of imagination to that of untruth, is part of the price we pay for our discursive control over our environment. If we can recover our imaginations it was probably worth paying, but in consequence of it there is a whole repertoire of biologically programmed human responses of which we make inadequate use or no use at all.

I should be inclined as a biologist to start the examination of the problem of literalism not from the word "religion" but from the conception of play—a non-serious activity which we allow to children and young animals, and occasionally to adults, in which literalism is suspended, mermaids can be assumed to be "real" for purposes of the game and children can be allowed (though not actively encouraged) to "believe" in them. Although we use the word of human activities in an undervaluing sense, it does in fact come rather closer to the sense of "emotional technology" than any other term. The thing we lack is a repertoire of non-reality-bound "games" which will involve release, controlled acting-out and a measure of consequent self-adjustment. Such games do not exclude extreme seriousness—there is a sense in which the devout Catholic "plays" that the host has become flesh, and primitive ceremonies which begin with boisterous and playful suspension of disbelief may end with extreme emotional exaltation.

We do not think of the French as particularly playful, but in this area their language is better equipped semantically than ours. In English the word *play* subsumes both *jeu (jeu sportif, jeux d'enfants)* and *pièce de théâtre*. We could with ethnological justification apply the word play to the enactments of the aborigines, of the child, of the theatre, of courtship, and of rituals public and private. Winnicott's concept of child play as a functional acting out, which may, properly managed, perform a "dream-work", is valid for all of these contexts. Much human emotional technology seems to involve what is phylogenetically a displacement activity, but one selected so that its content performs an emotional operation. There is still much argument how far aggressive play by children, and the acting out of violence in entertainment, are cathartic and how far they are incitatory to non-playful acting out. Fetishistic rituals are both similar to child play and at the same time examples of mini-theatre, enabling the actor-producer to deal with and partially circumvent anxieties by displacement—they are in other words part of *his* emotional technology, though the displacement does not get him any further with the task of handling the original sources of his anxiety. They are, however, quite clearly a programmed part of the whole spectrum of human reproductive behavior: though they are symptoms, if we saw them in certain individuals of a bird population we should call them adaptive. Indeed, if we set drama, child play, adult play, religio-magical ritual, sexual rituals and "hard-centered" activities like science and making money in a continuous row, there are few human activities, however purposive, which do not contain a play-element, often at the crudest level, as Genet so uncomfortably points out: we "play" at being bishops and even at being psychiatrists—it is very hard to be a soldier or a doctor without playing at being such.

The importance of this distinction between play and earnest is one of the linguistic and cultural manifestations of two-culture literalism. Religion and the Dream Time are play, whereas literal and discursive statements are earnest. In fact, by our acceptance of the dichotomy, we are actually less clear about the limits of fact and fiction than is the aborigine, and far more shamefaced in seeking pretexts to meet emotional needs. The citizen who dresses in a rubber suit to go skindiving is culturally justified—even if he does not go in the water: the citizen who is conscious of a desire to wear one on Saturday nights for sexual reasons he cannot verbalize is rather ashamed of the impulse and may, if other things upset him, consult a psychiatrist. A London purveyor of fetishistic paraphernalia, who defended himself against an indecency charge by saying that he only sold toys for adults, was speaking with some biological insight. Art and drama as vehicles for even unacceptable fantasy are near-respectable—religion is fully so, but the toys it has given us in the past are now within St. Paul's category of "childish things." At the same time, the word "play" does, for us, imply permission to relax, and in particular to relax the purposive and realistic mode of behavior. It would be worrying to some if we were to describe psychotherapy as a form of controlled play permitting such relaxation (less worrying, of course, if we say that some forms of art and of play are psychotherapeutic).

In one sense these phenomena are not "abnormal"—the human species is programmed for them as part of its equipment to offset infantile
Oedipal anxieties: what has been abnormal is the withering away of
the "emotional technology" by which an adjusted society accom-
modates some of them. One such technology is public ritualization;
comparable anxieties are comparably expressed in many "primitive"
rituals and in art. But from childhood this is the art of the individual.
As art has become a wholly individual and non-public activity, so
have these.

The individual medium for the psychodramatic expression of anxieties is *play,* which our culture confines to children. Compared with
the growing individualism of symbolic outlets which were classically
public—ritual, art and drama—play is expanding and attitudes to it are
loosening. The two processes are one, and art itself is becoming a form
of play as it comes to be bolder in open expression of unconscious
needs. Dress is a case in point. Stylized in most cultures at most times,
it is one of our most important ways of expressing either our public
image (in periods or occupations when it is conventional) or our real
selves, in periods when it is idiosyncratic. The Homburg-hatted gentleman is expressing the conformity of his image; the ringleaders of leath-
erwear and kinky boots express their own needs and anxieties—once
these have become general, swarms of followers use the same symbols
to indicate conformity to an image. But in fact, by putting on a Homburg
hat one is playing at being, not *a* businessman (which one is), but *the*
businessman. The child cannot at that moment be a nurse, or Batman,
or a police chief, but by putting on the clothes he can play at being
these real or fantasy people. The adult may express some at least of
the same inner material by *becoming* a nurse or a policeman, and the
interpenetration of real and fantasy, unconscious "play" and useful activity, is constant.

Where play is becoming more nearly, for us, what it might be adap-
tively is in the loosening of overall restraint on letting the unconscious
show—less for men than for women: a girl can now appear in thigh
boots and a Batman hood without being taken for a prostitute exhib-
iting a specialty, while a man can do so only by adopting a functional
excuse such as motorcycling or skindiving, thereby making play into
earnest. It is those most preoccupied with, or conscious of, the need
for such play—those whose potency depends on it, for instance—who
are least able to adopt such pretexts. We do not tolerate Shamans. Society demands a basic insincerity, typical of much fetishistic and similar fantasy; functionalism converts the play into earnest, and to some
extent spoils its magical function: except at a non-participant level in

the fantasies of films, television or comic books, which abound in fetishes, true play between adults acutely embarrasses and disturbs both the person who requires it (and is often anxious about it, which is why he needs it) and the culture. The really pathetic aspect of "deviant" journals devoted to minor fetishisms is the wish of the players for social support—the culture makes them play alone, even to the point of restricting their open association or search for partners for fear of encouraging "vice." Sometimes, through separation or even attrition, coupled with the capacity of a loving woman to mould her inclinations by conditioning, the game becomes happily two-sided and the secret a childhood secret which enhances the anxiety-discharging function of the game. But our social presuppositions do not encourage such comprehension. By keeping deviant needs secret they hinder assortation, and morality clamps down on public advertisement. This is something which indeed is getting better, partly through the advent of psychoanalysis, and partly through the general growth of personal frankness. But one still must be very driven to wish to be thought odd. Hence the pathetic resignation of the adult children in these fringe publications, always compelled to play alone, and excluded thereby from many of the emotional fruits of adulthood.

Sexuality is biologically the most important human form of play: this indeed, in an animal which mates when infertile and throughout pregnancy, represents statistically a greater part of its function than does reproduction. Part of this extension of mating into play clearly represents bonding behavior, but the human predisposition to sexualize almost all fantasy in the process of socializing it suggests a mechanism with other functions—an emotional technology analogous to our use of the dream seems at least a strong candidate for such a function. It is certainly true that anxiety-based rejections of sexuality overspill culturally into the rejection of playfulness, which is why the Protestant Puritan, with his intense distrust of the sub-adult and the pregenital, prefers stylized sport to unstylized—and hence dangerously revelatory—play. Even the play of Victorian children had to be edifying.

Probably the closest we have come to a prebiological notion of play as dream-work for adults is in Schiller's idea (The Aesthetic Letters) of play as the "abolishing of time in time"—of entry, in other words, into the Dream time. Its social and aesthetic fallout worried him, on the ground that Dionysian "playfulness" would lead to a release of repression and the "decay of higher values"—a point on which Marcuse[1] attempts to disabuse him. It is after all Dionysus, not primarily Apollo, who is the god of playacting: drama is the only aesthetic, however stylized, which is formally his preserve. A biologist would hardly, I think, pursue Bally's idea of creative play as representing a "space" where man for once is unbothered by his instincts—or if we prefer, his biological programming.[2] Whatever else is not evident about human—and sexualized—adult play, it is apparently programmed to perform some function as an adaptive character, and the programming is sufficiently precise in its canalization to make that function very probably specific. Notable among candidates for such possible contexts is the discharge of anxieties connected with dominance behavior: from the "motivational conflict" (a little like that in herring gulls) which makes the child initially confuse copulation with aggression, to the complex dominance behaviors involved in masculine and feminine role-playing, and the overriding dominance situation of Man, the relationship between parent and child in which the latter's mental processes already, through anticipation, seem to outrun his physical capacities. (Infantile sexuality, since it cannot in the nature of things be acted out, seems to predicate this.) A better appreciation of the human confusion between dominance and sexuality, which has obvious primate roots, clearly adds new overdeterminants to any attempt to expound sado-masochism.

The gratuitous playmate of early industrial society and earlier, was the professional prostitute. She provided the machinery through which some at least of the tension of solitariness and oddness was discharged from unusual heterosexual fantasy, and the brothel was an enclave of society where it was acceptable. This function was tension-relieving rather than therapeutic, but the same could be said of much psychotherapy. The institutional prostitute and her "house" are on the way out—humane moralism, which objected to a relationship, however stylized, overtly based on "use", has been more successful in banishing the professional than older moralisms based on a different dogma. In a sense this is right: where the fantasy is mutually realizable in an adult love-relation, the result for both parties can often be better. At the same time we may have sacrificed a valuable ritual convention for the wrong reasons.

This brings me back to the multiple meanings of the word "play" in English. Puritans were equally opposed to the brothel and to the stage, and tended to equate them. In both cases, some part of this hostility arose from fear of sexuality itself, and some part from fear of the exposure and realization of fantasy—non-seriousness. We could reword the diatribes of Roundheads against harlotry players in psychiatric terms. If we were Roundhead psychiatrists we would allege that both actress and whore are "handicapped" or "immature" people, whose problems lead them into role-playing.

In our own society, however, one is allowed fame and the other infamy, and the social valuation of the behavior involved determines the selection and quality of entry to the profession. In an imaginary culture where sexual playmates had a valued professional standing as psychagogues, girls might be advised by therapists to take up the occupation in order to act out profitably, and those who now enter it would have to find alternative ways of revenging themselves on parents or affronting society.

The analogy between the brothel and the theatre is insightful, at an intuitive level: both minister to fantasy, allow dressing-up and even crossdressing, involve ritual, and are concerned with play and plays—one recalls de Sade's theatricalism and interest in psychodrama, the Elizabethan boys playing girls playing boys, Justine as Goddess of Melodrama, the roots of drama itself in the rites of Dionysus—one could go on until shouted down by outraged actors and actresses. The fantasies of the brothel did, however, formerly differ from those of the theatre, not only in that the prostitute is exploited (actresses formerly were exploited, and prostitutes are so only because society insists upon it) but chiefly in that in the brothel "scene" the client both calls and enters into the drama. He, like the playwright, could determine, for once, the responses of others—as in a game with rules—and make them conform to his fantasy, a situation otherwise confined to, and very typical of, child play—"Now I'm a bear: you be the keeper and I'll eat you." This distinction, however, is getting blurred in some of the modern extensions of theater which encourage audience participation and improvisation. The professional cast here has exactly the function of the madame and her girls in the *divertissements* staged at Le Sphynx for Edward VII. At the private level of fantasy, for the less self-confident, one can now buy a record which enables one to play opposite a famous actress: or one in which a male masochist can hear himself reviled or ordered about by a female voice, with sound effects. I heard, in fact, of one resourceful fantasist in this genre who insulted himself before a tape recorder, and replayed the tape at a higher speed to simulate the female voice. Until recently our culture held the ring between such behaviors, by regarding it as intolerable that actual sexual activity should be presented on the stage. That is no longer the case.

I have been being deliberately perverse in this argument, not to devalue the theatre, but to indicate the real unity of human attempts at fantasy enactment. The real objection to bordel drama was that it was insightless—unlike the theatrical variety, it was tied to the stereotyped demands of anxiety (and boring to all who failed to share its commissioner's preoccupations), and we achieve nothing through it.

This can equally be true of anxious child play. The question is whether a therapeutic or self-knowing element could be injected into such psychodrama, not only if it were insightful, but also if play in a sexual context and with an *involved* and affectionate partner were in fact a biologically programmed part of human abreactive equipment—real play is with relationship, not with hirelings, as modern encounter drama recognizes.

Games involving aggression and sadism are those which cause us most cultural anxiety, both in adults and children. When children play them we rationalize this anxiety as fear of the mis-educative or addictive consequences—when adults do so we express a rational fear that someone may be hurt: both of these rationalizations, though substantial, cover our own sense of the inability of our culture to express sexual aggression acceptably and harmlessly. "No form of stimulation prior to coitus is wrong from the Christian point of view if both partners desire it and if it does not involve the personality-injuring cruelties of sadism and masochism."[3] Real cruelty is certainly a bad thing. On the other hand a largely symbolic interest in "cruel" play, punishment games and the like, which we tend to accept in children, probably finds a better adult expression in the ritual and sexual context, where it really belongs, than in diversion to other contexts where the cruelty becomes real. Presumably the acceptable standards for adults and for children are really alike. Nobody wants to encourage dangerous or painful behavior by either, but adults who play ritually at prisoners and torturers in the sexual context, embarrassed as our culture is apt to make them feel about it, do less harm than they would by providing excuses to do the same cathectic things in respectable earnest. In fact with mutual acceptance they presumably do none at all.

"Sex and violence" of this kind in private is a less difficult issue than its prevalence in entertainment. Here the drama in which we do not participate has virtual carte-blanche. What a rational pretext does for the fetishistic dresser-up, the requirements of "plot" or "seriousness" do for the dramatist. A lady may be buried alive or raped with a corncob if this is necessary to the serious intention of the work—but not, according to this view, simply for kicks. What humane and liberal criticism misses is that in literary composition—let us face it—the kicks and hokum come first. Throughout literary history melodrama and the comic book, hokum and sexual symbolism, are not grafted on "serious" art: they are the real powerhouse behind most of it, "seriousness" consisting in the skill and intellect with which talent develops these infantile and disreputable preoccupations. Nobody reading The Revolt of Islam can doubt whether the kicks or the literature came first: Shelley had no such doubts. Nor did Flaubert, for whom *Salammbô* was an "idée lubrique sans érection." Here the prudes have better intuition than the liberals. From this convention of double-think arises a second: that to play at flogging one's wife or husband is disruptive of public order and likely to make the tabloids, while to watch the innocuous flogging or combustion of a screen actress is disinfected—partially at least—because the fantasy is non-participant; besides, to see the same episode in a work of genius is actively uplifting. In my view the psychosexual material is identical in all cases. The play version has a personal fallout in tension-release, the "high class" literary version a fallout in the incidental communication of something worthwhile by way of emotional and cultural experience, and the Hollywood-Avengers version a possible fallout in the discharge of fantasy. At least it is a version of the anthropologically august habit of story-telling. All three can lead to trouble in borderline cases, and too much and too constant violence can indeed demoralize a culture. But I am inclined to look with less apprehension in all cases upon the play-versions of aggression than upon those which escape censorship through the convention of being in earnest—punishment, war, political violence and the like. The frontier we need to guard is not between love and aggression, but between sexual fantasy and spiteful reality. Meanwhile, in the acephalous world of censored entertainment one may represent aggressive behavior provided it is spiteful or criminal—one may tie up or wallop the heroine in order to rob her, but not with implications of love or sexuality; and the anxiety in this prohibition goes deeper than the reasonable observation that relatively few people of either sex enjoy being walloped in earnest as a manifestation of love.

Eissler[4] has made the point that the real aim of psychoanalysis is not only the removal of symptoms, but the complete reordering of human experience and if possible, the human condition. Mental disorders probably can be palliated by drugs, and even the capacity for insight might be increased by them, but our social and mental problems as a species might not be helped more by such desirable advances than they have been by antibiotics or surgery. There is no substitute, in other words, for insight and the capacity to feel and think, and it is these phenomena which psychoanalysis attempts to reorder. As a start, its particular approach and insight is the foundation for, or an ingredient of, all the new-look sciences of Man—against which naïve behaviorism or mechanism is simply out of date. To this extent it does look capable of providing not an ideology (these are usually deeply irrational) but an appropriate contemporary outlook, which is what religions have done in the past. By contrast with religions, however, modern "anthropic" science is the first opportunity we have had as a species of combining an awareness of emotional needs with the new and sophisticated rational empiricism. All that is in question—since such a synthesis is eminently what our culture needs—is our present capacity to take this and to find socially effective ways of implementing it. At least from now on insight will be as important to the physician (not to mention the judge or the businessman) as is discursive knowledge or empirical skill.

The biologist cannot regard the pregenital residues as "abnormal"—they are manifestly part of the natural history of the species. Sado-masochism, fetishisms and the like are displacement activities arising from, and compensating for, the Oedipal anxiety in the old primate family structure. They persist as part of human equipment because, though deleterious to some individuals, they have probably acquired social and displacement uses which paid off. Homosexual potentialities quite possibly enabled us to become functionally social, by giving the male group, which cuts across pair-mating family structure, the steam necessary for it to perform. In other words, these "abnormalities" are or were probably adaptive, at least as potentialities (that in large doses they upset reproduction is beside the point: social insects have evolved wholly sterile individuals). One cannot prove that the capacities for dominance-submission with pleasurable affect, or for erotic investment in objects, have been handholds in social evolution—a leather fetishist may have altered agricultural history by inventing the first horsecollar, or he may not—but to the biologist their commonness as human potentialities looks adaptive. It would be odd if so many of us were reproductively abnormal without some pay off.

It is only a hundred years since Krafft-Ebing catalogued every form of sexual behavior which he did not himself enjoy as a fully paid-up disease. A biological generation which is also psychoanalytically literate is bound to see that since most of the unscheduled sex behaviors are highly canalized—expressing, for example, displacement, interest in superskin textures, compression, skin and muscle eroticism, body image alteration, dominance-submission, or overdetermined mixtures of these—they have not only a psychosymbolism but also an ethology. In other words they are likely to be adaptive mechanisms, "put there on purpose"—and, as we would do if we saw comparable behavior in birds, we can ask, not "are they normal?" but "what are they for?" The insistence on genital primacy, the procreative view of sex, which is in Man, at least in the major part, a bonding and play behavior, and Puritan literalism probably have in common an anxiety-based rejection of many tunes which the human organ was programmed to play, for the better adjustment of our realistic relations; silence them here, and they appear as noises off, to our hurt. The attempt to discharge them by giving insight is arduous and not always successful—an ethologist would aim to see what constructive and insight- or adjustment-giving use could possibly be made of the psychodrama itself, since Nature appears to have laid it on. We use child play, since Winnicott, in this way, as well as to give clues to the therapist. The play groups of the future may well be—if they are not already—for adults.

References

1. Marcuse, H.: Eros and Civilisation. Boston, The Beacon Press, 1955, p. 192.

2. Bally, G.: Vom Ursprung und den Grenzen der Freiheit. Basel, Schwaber, 1945.

3. Hiltner, S.: Sex and the Christian Life. New York, Association Press, 1957.

4. Eissler, K.R.: Medical Orthodoxy and the Future of Psychoanalysis. New York, International Universities Press, 1965.

Deviation or Magic?

We have discussed sexuality as a vehicle for play, and play and theatre as safety-valves for the socialization of fantasy. Sexuality, our most playful and most unbuttoned activity, is the theatre designed by evolution or a benign Providence, according to how teleological we choose to get, for the enactment and civilization of some of these awkward intruders in a social animal. You will all quite easily spot these overdeterminants in conventional therapy with worried patients, and have the job of reassuring them and yourselves. At the same time, when behaviors look hostile and fantasies are alarming, one does have to consider just how much reassurance it is safe or ethical to give: somebody might get hurt. In drawing this line we encounter yet another overdeterminant and yet another use of sexuality, which is near-universal in human societies but which our society rather oddly discounts—the use of ordeal and of sexuality as magic.

There are two problems which confront any reasonably concerned and responsible author of a sex book—the first is what to put in and what to leave out; the second is what will be the likely social effects of the production. In turning what was to have been a treatise on ethology into The Joy of Sex we decided finally that we would include all nondangerous behaviors which appeared to be capable of use as resources rather than hangups. Sexuality itself, in its squarest marital manifestations, can be and is used to express neurosis, hostility and the like. So is excessive normality.

Maslow pointed out that there are no perverse behaviors, only perverse people. In other words, although sexual response is "canalized"—there is a limited repertoire of common releasers or turn-ons—it is always overdetermined, and whether a particular behavior is a problem-index depends on its place in the patient's lifestyle.

This is not the classical psychoanalytic position. At its most tolerant, classical therapy would recognize unusual or pregenital behaviors as symptomatic but sometimes egosyntonic and not necessarily to be disturbed. In a process of general psychic springcleaning such idiosyncratic "transitional objects" need to be addressed because of their diversionary potential. If the process is successful, they will lose their appeal, which will be transferred to simple in-out, in-out coition.

There are manifestly instances where this is true but, at the same time, the range of straightness shifts with social climate, and there is no sexual manifestation, including rigid insistence on genital primacy, which cannot be used to express personality difficulties. Strict Freudianism also misses the possibility that the very range of idiosyncratic human sexual behavior is adaptive, or "made a-purpose," to fit and to cushion the effects of our unique psychosocial development. This is almost certainly the case with our rooted potential for bisexual expression which may, when extreme, limit reproductive efficiency in some individuals, but also facilitates same-sex bonding. Our capacity for ritualization and fantasy is viewable as a displacement activity.

This more Panglossian view of the biological uses of behaviors is not typical of depth psychology, but needs integration into it. Freud, indeed, would hardly have committed himself to the doctrine of vaginal orgasm if he had considered that God would not have installed a doorbell if he had not meant it to be rung. The fact seems to be—again in Maslow's terms—that any rigidity in sexual preference, whether it be for a fetish or for the missionary position, is evidence of a potential or actual problem. Unanxious behavior drawn from a wide, personally appropriate repertoire correlates with high dominance, and it is possible that by increasing the range of the acceptable, which is one thing that books can undoubtedly do, one might actually go beyond mere reassurance to reduce neurotic emphases, rather as one can change attitudes by changing verbal behaviors. Mere withdrawal of social prescription can sometimes effect this. We now see "exclusive homosexuals" who, because of the withdrawal of the social prescription that one must be gay or straight but cannot be both, find themselves free for the first time to explore the heterosexual option without anxiety.

Pseudo-aggressive behaviors gave us most trouble, partly because in writing books one knows that the village idiot and the village psychopath are both listening, and partly because there is so much genuine spite in our society that even playful pseudo-violence is worrying. We accordingly talked to a great many self-styled "sadomasochists." We found a few whose sexual activities were genuinely masochistic and chimed with a lifestyle of social masochism and accident-proneness—a few genuine sadists likewise. We also found compulsive ritualists whose use of sex as a transitional object differed only from compulsive missionary-positionists in the repertoire to which they clung. Both of these groups could have done with therapy. We also found that for a substantial number of those who, having read psychiatric texts, admitted or boasted that they were "into S and M," sadomasochism ap-

peared to have little to do with it. The function of their exercise was
physical arousal, pretense of compulsion to overcome residual cultural blocks to letting-go, playfulness, and oddly enough—magic, the
use of ordeal to create oceanic sensation. We were in fact dealing with
would-be wizards, albeit on a domestic scale. Where anything was
being averted or appeased it was not so much guilt in regard to sex as
a far more atavistic sense of its dangerousness as a source of *mana*.

This was an unexpected overdeterminant, and it gives rise to some
interesting reflections on the dynamics of odd sexual choices and private rituals, based not on Krafft-Ebing but on Mircea Eliade's *Archaic
Techniques of Ecstasy*. Moreover, not only these particular emphases
such as restraint, chastisement, threat and external control of the
tempo of arousal, but others such as transvestism, homosexual expressions, the wearing of masks, and the cathexis attached to magical "protective clothing" of various kinds, which figure in idiosyncratic sexual
behaviors, figure also as religio-magical apparatus in a large variety of
cultures. In fact the playroom devised by one sexual hobbyist—what
an old-time French madam would have termed diplomatically *"un
specialiste"*—was depicted in a magazine for other specialists. It re-
called not the Inquisition but the *Magic Flute*. Having started to look
at sexual behaviors in terms of their natural history and their syntonic
and dystonic uses, we now had to look at their anthropology as parts
of an unspoken ethno-religious underground, a totally unforeseen
point of view.

Fortunately there was no need, in a counseling book, to go beyond
reassurance to those for whom unscheduled sexual behaviors "work."
The same would apply to most psychotherapy with those whom the
demands of the Spirits disturb. But the therapist might do well to think
of the religio-magical dimension simply because as a rule he does not
do so.

Religious interpretations of patient behavior are unusual in contemporary psychiatry which tends to be secularist even when it is, for example, Jungian. Moreover sexual experimentation is an improbable
venue for "religious" behaviors in the Judaeo-Christian tradition. To a
comparative anthropologist it would be less so, especially if we view
"religious" behaviors as including the range of oceanic experiences
which suppress the conventional experience of "I-ness" or homuncular identity. Three sexual modes are associated in anthropology with
the induction of oceanic, ecstatic, and similar mental states. One is the
sophistication of heterosexual intercourse by breath control, avoidance of orgasm and other techniques: the object here is to prolong the
"window" of partially dissociated or altered consciousness which im-

mediately precedes orgasm and to exploit it for yogic purposes. This is the leading exercise of Tantrik yogas. Another is sexual *koinonia*. "Open sexuality," though not widely practiced in statistical terms, is now quite widespread in Californian groups devoted to the development of "human potential." It is a widespread primitive expedient and features equally in left-hand Tantrik practice and among some semi-secret Krishna sects even in puritan modern India, and its antiquity is undoubted. It also, alone among our examples, has a history among American charismatic Christians such as the Adamites and the Agapemonites. Much of its effect is in the shock-value of deculturation, in "creative regression," or both. But Californians and others entering a secular *ras mandala* type experience out of curiosity or in pursuit of sexual "kicks" have on occasion found the anthropological efficacy of the rite disturbing in that the "hidden agenda" may indeed take over, and experiences of innocence, bonding, or disquieting self-confrontation may predominate over the salacious or the exciting, for which they originally came.

The third, and least complex, mode is *the use of ordeal* to acquire powers or to alter self-awareness. Now, ordeals are not normally sexual in a positive sense. In fact, abstention from sexual intercourse is perhaps the commonest in magico-religious practice. A person for whom sexuality involves, or appears to involve, ordeal is in our terminology a masochist, and with the religious associations of masochism our tradition is fully familiar. Unfortunately this association is interpretive, in that we read it as the use of ordeal or discomfort to atone for sexual guilt. This is not a feature of the widespread use of ordeal to manipulate consciousness in other traditions where another over-determinant, its use as an arousal technique to alter consciousness by a manipulation of the body image, is predominant. Of nondysfunctional couples who engaged in behaviors usually classified as sado-masochistic (command of one partner by the other, tying each other up, occasionally very mild pain infliction, and emphasis on what Reik calls the suspense factor), most appeared to be engaged in what was ethologically play, but others gave a strong impression of engaging in something very like yoga. In some of these couples a labored "aggressive" scenario introduced into the performance seemed to serve chiefly to reduce self-consciousness by making sense of an activity they did not fully comprehend in terms of psychiatric interpretations of such behaviors which they had read. People in our culture are acutely unhappy with significant experiences which they cannot classify. "Magic," in this context, would not be a socially acceptable explanation, but that is exactly how most anthropologists would classify such rituals if they were culture-approved, not self-invented.

Much has been written about the religious overtones of "masoch-ism," but chiefly in terms of asceticism. This is because our culture is familiar with ascetics who beat themselves to suppress sensual arou-sal, less so with ascetics who aim to enhance it or manipulate it for a religio-magical end. Although none of our nondysfunctional "sadoma-sochists" endured more than trivial discomfort, and all were unani-mous in rating actual pain as a downer, concentrating rather on ritualized body-image manipulation and heightened arousal by delay and a little mild "frightening," they struck us as being ascetics in the etymological sense—people who develop an askesis aimed at manipu-lating self-consciousness, even though the explanation they gave of their behaviors was that they found them physically exciting.

In nearly all archaic human traditions we find the concept of "or-deal" associated with the acquisition of magical powers. This use of "austerities" (self-testing, discomfort, infliction), expressed in Sanskrit by *tapasya* (the plural of tapas, heat) is not properly masochism, if by masochism we mean the pursuit of discomfort, pain or humiliation for its own sake. On the other hand it is arguable from observation that the overtly sexual masochist who needs to be flogged in order to reach orgasm, for example, is pursuing discomfort "for its own sake." In most instances he is not. We have tended to look, in both the religious and the sexual context, to self-punitive motives, and in both cases they are not rarely present, at least as original sources of the notion behind the behavior. It could equally be true that there are athletes who un-dergo extreme *tapasya,* and would-be astronauts who volunteer for dangerous and unpleasant training, rather to propitiate inner guilt than because of the effects on performance. Yet, the performance may justify the rationalization. The point is that *tapasya* of the traditional kinds prescribed respectively for sexual, mystical or athletic purposes produce effects on performance and experience in these fields *per se* which transcend the conscious or unconscious object which led an in-dividual to adopt them. Thus, wholly penitential flagellation can pro-duce embarrassingly secular orgasm, and people whose motives in undertaking ascetic or masochistic exercises were probably sexual may find themselves experiencing altered consciousness of a non-sex-ual character.

Religious ordeals are unpopular in our culture, as we are shocked by the notion that boot camp produces better soldiers. In fact athletic per-formance and sexual arousal are now the only settings in which we can observe the specific effects of *tapasya* without being made uncom-fortable about them—a striking reversal.

"Masochism" in its sexual context is so heavily overdetermined, involving physical stimulation, elements drawn from general dominance-behaviors and carried over into sex, and concepts built on infantile ideas of guilt and punishment at the Freudian level, that most psychiatrists would be glad to drop it altogether, distinguishing "programmed plays" (which heighten sexual arousal), anxiety-appeasing rituals which act as transitional objects, in the manner of a teddy bear or a beloved piece of blanket, and genuinely self-destructive behaviors. The trouble is that any or all of these may coexist, so that one man's playfulness is another man's disability. Something very similar applies to the masochisms of the religious—what started as pathological self-punishment may unexpectedly lead to religious rather than sexual arousal, and what has been taught by *sadhus* as a means of heightening religious arousal (abstinence, discomfort, sensory deprivation, and *tapasya* generally) will naturally appeal to the pathologically anxious and self-punitive whether or not they lead to fusional experience. Add to this that sexual arousal is fusional, though not all fusional experiences are sexual, and we come the full circle and can enter the continuous performance at any point. It is all very complicated. What is clear is that if many serious *sadhus* engage in masochistic-looking austerities, they do not do it for kicks, or not for the same kicks as the "masochist"—though one variety of kick is in certain respects linked to the other.

One is tempted to see asceticism as a purely cultural outgrowth of the mystical undertaking and pathological at that, being based on the fact that those who most fear their own I-ness most want to get rid of it, but askesis does not necessarily involve masochism, and the testimony is fairly unanimous, even among those who reckon that their exercises no more than facilitate, rather than reliably produce, changes in I-experience. Thus even frankly orgiastic yogas enjoin discipline of a negatively reinforced kind, and even avoid orgasm in the specific mystical use of sexuality, though this is rationalized physiologically as "conserving semen." It may be that the negatively reinforced "I" can be treated like a phobia and "flooded" by pushing negative reinforcement or frankly aversive inputs to a point where the system breaks down. Couple this with the disorienting effect of *tapasya* such as fasting, immobility and sensory deprivation, and the ascetic recipe begins to make sense. It is not a necessary condition of unconventional "I" perception any more than is the taking of LSD, but those who have practiced it—like the masochist Heinrich Suso quoted by William James—from quite other, and probably sexual, motives, found empirically that altered I-states followed. The bizarre recipe for aversive self-treatment given by St. John of the Cross passes with agility from "seeking that which is most distasteful" to a validly mystical formula ("So as to be all things, be willing to be nothing") and from thence into diction prefiguring what sounds very like orgasm, a sequence which gives us some of the operants of the *nirvikalpa* mode of perception, though not yet the exact roles which they play. Evidently it can be triggered by austerity, or by displaced sexuality, the two reinforcing each other in some mystics as many non-mystics. Indeed, there are few of the physical dodges and attacks on the body image which are used to achieve magical or mystical states which are not also used by some people and traditions to achieve the secular mystical experience of heightened orgasm.

In our society, charismatic and initiatory yogas directed to sexual ends constitute the only spontaneous magico-religious rituals of I-manipulation which we can observe. It might still seem odd to classify the sexual rituals of so-called sadomasochists as "religious," but their anthropological relation to traditional magic is close. So far it has usually been studied from the wrong end (by classing magical operations as sadomasochistic) rather than by treating purported sexual rituals as genuinely magical—a distortion which the participants often promote by adopting the common psychiatric valuation of their behaviors and enacting charades in conformity with it.

The relationship of the manipulating or "top" partner to the manipulated or "bottom" partner, when we actually observe it, belies that content of the charade which may be played. It is not in fact that of dominator or master to dominated or slave, but that of facilitator of psychopomp, who uses control to evoke, to push into transcendent experience—almost exactly that of coach to athlete or platoon commander to recruit. Like the coach or the commander, the manipulator "compels" the manipulated into states or performances of which the manipulated did not know themselves to be capable, but the compulsion is skillful facilitation, since the states evoked represent only the expression of potentials already present. Often the only function of the charades is to give coherence and superficial meaning to the "game," which is exactly analogous to any other training-game depending on evocation and psyching-out the trainee, who may be in the event, experientially enhanced, not humiliated, by the total experience. In reality the "top" partner is psychologically the more passive, since he or she appears to act as an externalized projection of the "bottom" partner, or some component of their identity actively externalized, an extraordinary form of reified transference. The embodiment of externalized selves for the use of others—the clients or initiates—is a conventional but neglected role both of the shaman or initiator and of the psychotherapist; this is one of its most striking modern forms. That the ritual is in this case sexual and the overt objective sexual arousal is in line with our lack of dissociative experiences outside the sexual field, but as with so many overtly sexual experiments ("open" or group sexuality being another), there is a hidden agenda which is not sexual so much as magical or magico-religious, and which tends to take over.

This ethological interpretation is not so far at variance with the Freudian view as might appear. The charade overtly or covertly includes reminiscences of punitive individuation, and the recapitulation of these in order to "get behind" them facilitates the recreation of a pregenital, non-individuated experience. In magic, however, as opposed to symptomatic sadomasochism, ordeals represent not a continuing appeasement of guilt by infliction, but rather a form of initiation or ongoing rite de passage. The singularity of this, compared with other more social rites de passage, is that it is a backward-running initiation, into pre-Oedipal experience. Merlin, the chief yogic wizard of Celtic tradition, was born an old man and died an infant, a highly significant myth. In shamanic traditions "acting backwards" is a source of magical power, beside being a denial of the unidirectionality of Time, which in oceanic states looks like a structural consequence of the mechanics of I-ness. The naive masochist who is turned on by being treated as a baby undergoing the aversive phase of individuation may accordingly be onto an anthropological and magical maneuver of greater power than he realizes.

If one in fact examines rather than psychoanalyzes the actual practices of people who—in the modern climate of public sexual confession—profess themselves to be "into S and M," one will find that these commonly have very little to do with either one, and a great deal to do with body-image manipulation. They are using ordeal as a means of altering identity boundaries—in this case pursuit of sexual orgasm at a heightened level—physical restraint, sensory deprivation, postponement, mild pain and occasionally an element of fear. These techniques are precisely those used traditionally in shamanic arousal, but guilty people will also use them in expiation, and self-destructive people as a means of self-mischief. Reich's percipient view of the masochist as one who wants to transcend or explode the body image—to burst, in fact—and who may assault the boundaries of the actual body in doing so, applies almost equally partly to the mystic, who wishes to implode the illusion of identity. The ego being a body ego, attacks on the body image seem to be built-in to this process physiologically and the ordeals imposed on themselves by those whose motives, like those of St. Simeon Stylites, were almost certainly self-punishing at a psychoanalytic level may in fact produce the other types of experience for which nonpathologic mystics undertake them. In Roman society, where overt pathologic sadism was an institutionalized public entertainment, the singular ordeal of the Villa of the Mysteries with its frightened and flagellated initiate exhibits the other use of such apparently punitive behaviors.

Indeed, we can go further and recognize in genuine sadomasochism the pathological misreading of the magico-sexual use of "ordeal," which interprets it as hostility in the service of anxiety and guilt, and expresses that hostility in sexual cruelty. To the legitimacy of magic directed at the body-image it opposes a sorcery which attempts to hijack or force the magic in mitigation of personal insecurity and disturbance. This closely resembles the child's misreading of the "primal scene," where vigorous coition is read as a hostile act, and hostility may be attached to the concept of the sexual or of love itself. De Sade and Gilles de Rais were such misguided sorcerers; the truly punishing or self-punishing saints, the sore-covered ascetics and flagellants, and the Inquisitors, represent the religious wing of this deviation. We can learn more of this interaction from J. K. Huysmans, perhaps, than from a psychoanalysis which, like the child seeing its parents in coition, misses the legitimate significance of behaviors which have a biology; such analysis draws its interpretation from patients who similarly misread them and endanger themselves and others in consequence. Masochists may assault the body-image but attempts to manipulate the body-image amounting almost to assault are not a sufficient criterion of masochism. We see them in the athlete, the lover, and the mystic also.

References

1. Comfort A: The "Normal" in Sexual Behavior. J Sex Educ Therap 2:1-7, 1975.

2. Comfort A: Homuncular Identity-Sense as a Deja-vu Phenomenon. Brit J Med Psycho 50:313-314, 1977.

3. Eliade M: Shamanism: Archaic Techniques of Ecstasy. New York: Bollingen Foundation, 1964.

4. James W: The Varieties of Religious Experience. 1903.

5. Maslow AH: Self-esteem (dominance-feeling) and Sexuality in Women. J Social Psychol 16:259-280, 1942.

III

On Sexual Problems

A Return To Kinsey

In spite of Freud, we go on in our assessment of science playing the old charade. Artists have unconscious motives, scientists are detached and presumably have none, either in choosing science as a field of activity and a general approach to experience, or in picking their topic. Scientific writers on sex and scientific students of sexual phenomena are more than ordinarily free of personal involvement, and sharply distinguished from the voyeur, the pornographer, the man with problems. So is the doctor, pinstripe or white coat.

Like most nonsenses, this one has a function. We distrust our own judgment so much, and so rightly, on topics which involve us deeply, that for dispassionate study to be possible we have to invent the perfect observer as we invent the perfect gas. In our own rational research we have to approximate our behavior to that standard, though unless we are deeply ignorant of psychology we shall also seek, and be helped rather than hindered by, insight into our own deep involvement, whether it be with sexuality or molecular behavior.

The cover story of the dispassionate observer has no possible support in the history of human biology. Darwin and Freud owed their achievements to the capacity to check their intuitions factually, but they owed their intuitions to their unconscious needs, and the combination accounts for their success in penetrating our cultural armor. Sexual studies are the field in which this process is the most obvious. Such studies are promoted by people who are motivated to the point of eccentricity, or they would never have involved themselves in so alarming an adventure. The gurus of sex are not the unconcerned, but those, like Havelock Ellis, Marie Stopes, Charles Bradlaugh, or Kinsey, who are involved to the point of near-eccentricity, but can deal with their involvement only by making it rational.

Kinsey, like Freud, has become synonymous in our minds with the sexual revolution. That there is an almost complete failure of communication between their findings is really inherent in what I have been saying, for the Kinsey approach almost excludes psychoanalytic insight. This is unimportant for the result, for we can put the two together. In 1937 a professor of zoology in Indiana turned his attention to the straightforward statistical description of human sexual behavior in his culture—he was prompted by the fact that he could not answer simple factual questions from students and colleagues about the prevalence of various sexual experiences, but it can hardly be a secret that he was equally concerned to answer questions about his own experience. Until his death he continued with skill, persistence, ingenuity, bloodymindedness and charm to collect interview data on all those aspects of sexual life which had previously been dealt with by guesswork, folklore or plain invention. He was something of a tyrant, a brilliant organizer, and a publicist of genius. A man who could meet irate Roman Catholic mothers and send them away convinced that by interrogating their daughters he was helping the health and virtue of the human race can do almost anything, and Kinsey did it.

He was helped throughout by the early discovery of transference—that interrogation about people's problems is tantamount to an offer of help. Jeremiahs who predicted that people would either tell him lies or show him the door were proved wrong by the immense wish of the ordinary American to know the truth about himself, get help in overcoming the isolation which reticence imposed on sexual experience in the old dispensation, and help others at the same time. Endless ammunition has been fired at Kinsey's statistical methods and volunteer-selection procedures, much of it blank, and all of it off-target. The important breakthrough was not in ascertaining the exact frequency of what the survey hideously calls "total outlet," or the wide prevalence of supposedly unacceptable behaviors, but in getting the American world to accept that such facts were ascertainable, and that when ascertained they made nonsense of the entire cultural fiction.

The surveys were non-evaluative: that is to say, the massive best-sellers in which they were published—ponderous and often pompous treatises which couldn't be faulted on public appeal but sold like hot cakes to people who could not read a graph—fell over backward avoiding any hint of approval or disapproval in their text. At the same time, the very statement that this is how people live in fact, as opposed to cultural fiction, has evaluative overtones for a world brought up on commandments. It makes one ask if the commandments were realistic in the first place, and there was no prize for the answer.

At the scientific level, Kinsey's team come nowhere near to a biologically complete account of human sexual behavior even in a single culture, for symbolic behaviors and the significance of individual patterns of preference, over which the studies were as silent as over desirability, account for a huge part of human ethology. There was a block incorporated in the original conception against becoming aware of these significances, and the block could be rationalized as factual sobriety and the avoidance of speculation. The issue of *normality* is central to a statistical study. Kinsey avoided the word—his concerns are with prevalence and with scatter (a favorite word of approval to an interviewee, I am told, was "you're way out on the tail of the distribution..."). We get no hint of the functional roles of supposedly abnormal behaviors such as homosexuality or fetishism in the evolved behavior of the species as a whole—almost certainly such apparently unadaptive things had functions for society, in maintaining the male group or stimulating human object-interest, but such Darwinian and biological ideas of the normal never appear. Still less do we encounter the $64,000 question in' psychiatric evaluation: "what does this behavior mean to *this* person?" Enough that it occurs in eight persons out of ten.

It is easy to bridle at this incompleteness, but the importance of the result is not really diminished. Krafft-Ebing had listed every form of sexual activity he could find which he did not himself practice, and had classed these as abnormalities; Kinsey simply listed them and showed them to be common. Some of the things so demythologized must, one feels sure, be commoner still if sought for in the right way— minor fetishes or sadomasochisms, for example, to judge by the content of fantasy expressed. The painstaking avoidance of significance in sexual behavior also seems to have behind it an overconcentration on the purely mechanical—how big, how many, how often. This is a disease of our outlook, but for this reason it can also be a therapy. Masters and Johnson have lately found that bringing sexual experience into the laboratory and treating it in terms of crude mechanics can help anxious Americans—the patients come from a culture far more used to manipulating things than handling emotions, and the acceptance of sexuality as a physical act removes it from the dark side of the moon to a sphere of acceptance and comprehension where its emotional side can be dealt with preconsciously. The Kinsey formula, like the Masters formula, is tailored to a machine culture, but none the worse for that—machine cultures need to be approached through concepts and experiences they can understand.

It is sometimes asked how much feedback such a highly publicized survey has produced in giving a sense of permission to waverers. Kinsey thought that it did not, because of the extreme rigidity of sexual patterns of preference once established, but I would like to see figures. The craw-thumping of the righteous over adolescent promiscuity is said by Schofield[1] to have made some previously unanxious youngsters wonder if they were missing something, and statistics bear hard on those who come below the median. In a curious way, Kinsey's university background accurately reflects a cultural neurosis which turns up repeatedly in the attitudes of patients—sexuality is like a competitive examination, in which grades are given and scoring matters, and it is among the examinee class that anxiety over "fulfillment" is possibly highest. In the mechanization of a personal relationship and in this scoring concept we have two irrational cultural attitudes highly typical, I suspect, of modern America and possibly modern Britain. Just as Kinsey's own preoccupations were turned to good use in his work, so were those of his culture and age. I know of no other way that man can be studied. We must work with the material we have, and a mechanistic age must use methods proper to itself, at least in the cover-story it puts up. The rest of the work of selfknowledge can still go ahead at other levels, while our attention is diverted.

It is interesting to contrast Kinsey with the founding father of sexual enlightenment, Havelock Ellis. Ellis was almost pathologically shy, despite his public courage, and collected nearly all of his data by letter—a most dangerous expedient in this field, where even the sex assumed by a letter-writer may be fantasied. The quality of his published case histories indicates a striking flair on Ellis's part for the empathic detection of the genuine. I never had the privilege of meeting Kinsey, but by contrast with Ellis he appears from the written record curiously naive—a grave handicap in the speculative student of human behavior. Only a naive man could have written of coital posture that "in view of the lack of evidence that any of these positions have any mechanical advantage in producing orgasm...they must be significant primarily ...as psychological stimulants." True, but there are also only two tunes, loud and soft. One wonders if the man ever *had* intercourse. I saw evidence of a similar unworldly attitude in some of the Institute's documentation—I think it was Kinsey's own attitude, for his successors and collaborators are and have always been pretty hardheaded. One "handwritten" letter in a female hand offering photographs for sale was in fact photolithographed like a highclass begging letter, and some credulity seemed to hang over the collection of large sexual-experience diaries submitted by volunteers. Ellis would have known by feel which were fact and which fantasy, and would have got it right on most occasions. At one time pornographic matter was being produced expressly for sale to Kinsey.

Having said all this, however, the solidity of the achievement remains. After all, the data were collected and are there, and if we dislike the analysis we can analyze it in our own way. Law enforcement agencies, the U.S. Customs, the Universities, the Church—all of them, by the end of his life, were eating out of Kinsey's hand. No previous investigator had this kind of cooperation from the thorniest and most disturbed of his fellow citizens. Kinsey managed to talk professional purity crusaders into supporters. Even prisons gave up their graffiti. Among pioneers of unpopular rethinking, Kinsey was unique in his capacity for not upsetting people—Ellis was prosecuted, Freud abused; only Burton was knighted, and he crept up on Victorian England in Oriental disguise. Kinsey went in by the front door.

Institutes of "sexology" are a necessary evil in the face of the clandestinity, fantasy, and anxiety attached to sexual documentation, and the steady and often rapid loss of important ephemera which do not get into libraries. Ideally they should be attached to departments of human biology in general—so that ethology, psychoanalysis, physiology and cultural anthropology all have a share. Kinsey came no closer to this than a department of zoology, and the exclusions implicit in this are symbolic. The material once collected, however, the interdisciplinary possibilities remain. Failing a proper study of man in depth—which in this field means combining Bloomington, Masters' institute, the Tavistock and the Max Planck Institut, so far as reproductive and psychosymbolic man is concerned—we might do worse than copy the Kinsey model in Britain where there is no comparable collection. I commend the possibility to the newly-formed Havelock Ellis Society. The British like to think of themselves as "less naive than the Americans and less cynical than the French"—a British institute might or might not confirm the cultural fiction, but it is certainly needed.

Yet another limitation in Kinsey's work, which was no fault of his team or of himself, since both tried hard to achieve completeness, was in the extent to which they appear culture-limited. Bibliographies are enormous and pains were taken to include in the background, if not in the studies, Japanese and other material which happened to come to hand. The oddest omission, to an Englishman brought up in the Ellis tradition, is the relative unawareness of Greek and Roman culture. This is important because the teaching of the Classics has been one of the few informational and reassuring palliatives upon English upperclass—and by extension American—sexual attitudes. Sanskrit and Islamic cultures did not touch us until Burton, tribal cultures only with the advent of cultural anthropology and psychoanalysis. If none of us had been able to read Juvenal, Martial and Petronius our cultural anxieties might have been even deeper. Contact with another culture's literature in depth was one of Havelock Ellis's greatest strengths. Modern American studies attempt to recoup this lack through anthropology (often with odd results, since urban Greece and Rome are more directly relevant to our own behavior than the Trobrianders)—Ford and Beach,[2] for example, miss the major literature-producing cultures, all of which give spectra of sexual behaviors very close in range if not in detail to those which emerge from the American surveys. This is a respect in which a British institute—if they are fairly quick about it, before technocracy blots out the characteristically double and amateur background of British biologists—could score, and in which the Arts man scores as a member of any team investigating human behavior. We are in a posture to continue Kinsey's work and extend it in a way that he—as a wasp man, not an Arts man, with the psychological choices which that implies—would have found difficult. At the same time, without his initiative we would not be in that posture today.

Neither Kinsey nor Ellis was in fact a physician, but they have had a profound influence on medicine, because we practice in a post-Kinseyan world. Their achievement has been to adjust our vision of sexual reality. Patients, even if they have not read them, are influenced in their expectation by the vortices these authors have left in modern society. Our patients are less bothered about compulsive normality and more inclined to take a prosaic view of oddities which, they now know, they share with thousands of fellow humans. Psychiatry has been bothered about Kinsey's reductionism—after all, sexual styles are a part of personal styles: they reflect early conflicts—they involve acting-out. But when it was the accepted wisdom only a few years ago, that all "homosexual" persons were paranoid, or at least deeply disturbed, there is a salutary corrective in recognizing that all humans have bisexual drives, that all "heterosexual" persons have homosexual fantasies. A moral preoccupation was being translated, as it so often has before, into terms of pathology in order to camouflage the translators' anxieties.

This is where the fact that Kinsey and Ellis started from human natural history scores. It is not a denial of the importance of "feelings," but in a psychiatric tradition which was encouraging us to keep feelings as pets—to pamper and overfeed them, and to take them regularly to the veterinary practitioner—they were and are a valuable counterpoise. We need to avoid excessive reductionism in viewing the new role in which we are cast as sexual counselors, but at least we can now do so with a roughly accurate idea of the prevalence of behaviors which patients described with an anxiety springing from the conviction that such problems are bizarre or unique, but which may statistically not be problems or indices of pathology at all.

References
1. Schofield, M.: The Sexual Behavior of Young People. London, Longmans, 1965.

2. Ford, C.S. and Beach, F.A.: Patterns of Sexual Behavior. London, Eyre and Spottiswoode, 1952.

Primary care for sexual problems

It is generally agreed that most primary physicians make poor counselors on sexual problems, but that they *could* sex counsel well and are probably the most appropriate individuals to do so. They have done it badly because of several factors: lack of research knowledge coupled with a medical literature based on folklore, lack of instruction in medical school, and possibly even psychologic causes connected with the selection of medicine as a profession—causes that make the physician "uptight" about sexual matters.

These things are now being remedied by a process of cultural change. Today the main bars to good sex counseling by the family doctor are time pressure and the absence of specific how-to instruction. Unlike other problems of patients, sexual difficulties may not be volunteered—one gets experience in treating them primarily by being the sort of person whose verbal and nonverbal communication with the patient makes him or her willing to volunteer them. With today's greater openness about sexuality, physicians can expect to deal with patients who talk without embarrassment about orgasm or erection.

Most sexual problems are "psychologic," and accordingly, if one doesn't know precisely how to handle them, there is the temptation to refer—in this case to the psychiatrist. True, many sexual problems reflect the whole style and personality of the patient and longstanding difficulties such as impotence produce disproportionate anxiety and disturbance. On the other hand, most such symptoms are also "functionally autonomous," that is, whatever their psychodynamic origins they are often easily removed, *as symptoms,* by relatively simple measures. (Almost all anorgasmic women, for example, can learn to experience orgasm, and it is easier to teach them than to provide them with new marriages or new personalities. Quite a few may prove to have not "inhibitions" but high blood prolactin levels.)

When this is done, the removal of a symptom that has often overhung the patient's whole lifestyle is at worst immensely reassuring, even if it releases new problems, and at best can open him or her to new insights without a great deal of therapy. By contrast, the more traditional idea that the therapist should ignore symptoms and go for root causes, aside from exposing the patient to long and expensive treatment, risks reinforcing the symptom habit, if only by duration: at worst one could have 10 years of psychotherapy, acquire much self-knowledge, and stay impotent.

The six problems

An accessible and confidence-giving family doctor ordinarily will encounter six common sexual problems, and others occasionally. These are the common ones:

1. **Fear or conflict over masturbation** is still surprisingly present in both sexes after a generation of reassurance. The ready acceptance of orogenital techniques as healthy and normal in many American marriages possibly has something to do with the idea that one should not touch the genitalia with the hands. The idea that past masturbation may have something to do with many other dysfunctions is almost universal, if only as an occasional doubt. Thus, reassurance in the form of direct endorsement is the key to dealing with this problem. A great many patients with sexual problems would benefit from being taught to masturbate frequently by prescription. The thing the physician must avoid is the projection of his own anxieties and doubts by the use of cop-out words like "in moderation" or "if not excessive." The anxiety-seeking patient will pick up these clues.

2. **Body image** problems are commonly seen as anxiety over penile size, breast configuration, or the effects of circumcision or uncircumcision—the specifically sexual manifestations of a general symptom pattern that extends to obesity, feelings of ugliness, and the demand for plastic surgery. If straight reassurance and the conversational attempt to show the patient that his or her dissatisfactions represent diffidence about the self and not a part of the body do not remove the anxiety, refer the patient to the psychiatrist and not the plastic surgeon. Penises that really are small, major endocrine dysfunction apart, cannot be enlarged but function well in every respect except as dominance signals. Breasts that are uncomfortably large and faces that really are grotesque can be improved by surgery. Remember that the body image cannot be so easily modified, however; so guard against the psychologic overlay that makes you, rather than a crooked nose, responsible for ruining the patient's life. In some instances operation on clitoral or penile phimosis is worth doing, but whether its effects are rational or magical is unclear.

3. **Impotency and premature ejaculation.** Greater than 90 per cent of

secondary impotency (that which occurs in a man who has been potent) is psychogenic and caused by anxiety over sexual performance. Age has little or no physical effect in precipitating it, except in the case where an aging man has discontinued all sexual activity, e.g., during the serious illness of a wife, and may then have difficulty in restarting. The common physical precipitants of impotency are overstress, diabetes, obesity, and alcohol, including alcohol in small or moderate quantities and especially when it is used to relieve performance anxiety. In such cases, one drink in some individuals can turn off performance and initiate a vicious circle. If an individual ever gets an erection (on waking, on masturbating, and so on), obviously nothing is wrong with the hydraulics. Testosterone alone is rarely deficient; in the view of some investigators it can be used to lower the threshold of erectility, but its use in the first place does more to reinforce the notion that something is physically wrong than to overcome the patient's problem. Anxious impotency of recent onset can—and should—be dealt with before it becomes a habit by reassuring the patient and by reducing the pressure of performance. The eminent 18th century surgeon John Hunter did this by telling the patient to continue sleeping with his anxiety-producing partner but forbidding intercourse for six weeks. The patient could not remain abstinent. Temporary abstinence from alcohol removes the problem in some men.

Yet if impotency continues, the physician should counsel the couple in the ways described by Masters and Johnson and simultaneously provide general sex education. Many men, for example, are unaware that there are unerectile modes of love play that satisfy a woman and direct attention away from the goal of performance. A physician can easily learn these psychotherapeutic skills, but since impotence is a self-aggravating habit and the skills of dealing promptly with it need training to acquire, there is a case for early referral. It needn't be to a psychiatrist as first resort, unless there are other gross problems, but to a sex therapist or clinic (if one is available) or to a behavioral therapist. Diabetes, undiagnosed depression, and the effects of prescription drugs and endocrine dysfunction should be excluded before referral.

Premature ejaculation is a larval form of impotence. The initial advice, by way of trial, is that the subject repeat intercourse as soon as he can get an erection (normally within minutes). If this fails to work and the erection to materialize, the next step is to counsel both partners, instructing them in non-demand love play leading to the squeeze technique. This is best done with films or tapes, which are available. In sophisticated couples, results are easily obtained. If the doctor himself is sophisticated but the partners are not, he may be unprepared to handle the shock induced by the suggestion that the woman handle her husband's penis, and a great deal of undergrowth may have to be cleared before any simple therapy can have a chance.

Where behavioral therapy is available, it can attack impotency by anxiety discharge or by use of biofeedback to teach voluntary control of erection. Its major advantage is that results, if they are going to be obtained at all, will be obtained quickly. If this approach fails, full psychiatric referral always remains. Behavioral therapy also can be useful to handle secondary consequences of symptom removal, such as when the cure of one partner's impotence induces frigidity in the other, or vice versa.

4. **Frigidity in women** is generally classified by most workers into orgasmic and preorgasmic types on the grounds that there is no jungle so thick that one cannot hack one's way through it. Women may remain preorgasmic through the couple's incompetence and lack of enterprise; through unwillingness to "give" to a particular person, or at all; through basic distaste for sexuality; through more complex causes; or a mixture of all these. In a couple with a good relationship and a reasonably enterprising sex life, the anorgasmic woman does best if provided with a program of "homework" in which she learns body exploration, self-stimulation, and transfer of her responses to the partner situation. Women who are orgasmic to oral and manual but not to vaginal stimulation can learn in most cases to respond to all three modes. Still, they need to lose the anxiety that motivates the request for therapy before they can respond. This type of behavioral therapy is again well within the scope of the family physician, but it takes time and needs to be learned. Once again, and for the same reasons, the first referral is to a sex therapist or a behavioral therapist.

5. **Vaginismus** is a related body image disorder, expressed in extreme spasm, and often leads to long-standing failure to consummate sexual relations. It can be treated by a similar homework schedule of graded desensitization—relaxation, self-insertion of graduated dilators, insertion of these devices by the partner, and finally, insertion of the penis.

Strange sexual behaviors
6. The only other commonly volunteered sex problem concerns **unusual behaviors,** or behaviors the patient regards as unusual, from regular parts of the repertoire such as orogenital contacts through optional preferences (minor fetishes, fantasy-type sexual play) to major sexual obsessions or socially disabling behaviors such as exhibition-

ism. The first of these calls for simple reassurance and some instruction in the variety of human sexual needs to both partners, one of whom may be showing extreme anxiety over his or her spouse's "perverted" or "sick" preferences. Books can help here. The last, major sexual obsessions, calls for psychiatric referral, depending on the physician's own willingness to judge between the need for depth psychology and the likely efficacy of "crash" behavioral methods in damage control. Most physicians will prefer to leave this choice to the psychiatrist.

"Homosexuality" or, rather, patient anxiety about it, has not been a common office complaint, but greater openness is making it so. It is a field where the physician who shares the gender anxiety common to his culture has to guard against expressing it. All humans possess the options of homosexual and of heterosexual response. Most show a predominant use of one of these, although the other may emerge unexpectedly in an unfamiliar context or under pressure and cause great alarm. The relative influences of learning and of physical and cultural determinants in directing the choice are not yet understood.

In dealing with patients who consult about this, the task is to correct cultural miseducation about what constitutes perversity, vice, and unworthiness. The aim, especially in young people going through a homosexual "trip," is to conserve their options and reinforce them against the cultural pressure to join one of two imaginary camps for life. Older patients who are upset by surfacing homosexual needs basically require information about the generality of such potentials and reassurance that they are not becoming "queer." The physician, however, should be on the lookout for the patient in whom disturbance of habitual gender identity heralds the start of a major psychosis or depression.

Since having homosexual potentials is not a disease, it can no more be cured than can heterosexuality. The individual who has acquired a habit and lifestyle of homosexual expression, who wishes to change or supplement it, needs not to lose the response to his or her own sex but to acquire the skill of relating equally or preferentially to the other sex—by overcoming both Freudian and socially reinforced anxieties. Behavioral therapy based on reinforcement, not aversion, succeeds well when the postulant has some heterosexual experience to reinforce. It is best done by experts. The physician's role as counselor turns on freeing himself from the judgmental folklore of the past, overcoming any anxious distaste he may have for potentials he himself has repressed, and helping his patient to do likewise.

The practitioner's choice

It should be evident from these notes that the doctor's choice about
how far he will engage in practical sex problem therapy, the point at
which he will refer, and to whom he will refer depends on the time he
is willing to devote to acquiring skills and practicing them. As a minimum he should be able to deal with reassurance and first-aid or first-
trial expedients and should present the face of an unembarrassed,
nonjudgmental, and sexually positive listener. If he is willing to acquire the relatively simple skills needed for second-instance therapy,
he will solve a major problem—the paucity of good sexual therapy in
many places and for many income groups while dubious and sometimes unskilled "therapy" abounds. By far the best way of acquiring
not only the skills of dealing with specific problems but also the attitudinal or "existential" background of self-awareness and body
awareness that will enable him to emphasize what the patient feels, or
lacks, is to go himself through a course of discussion, couple counseling, and instruction with peers under a competent therapist. Some
medical schools now provide this training, and it could be more
widely organized for established practitioners. One or more group
practices could organize such an experience for themselves, with the
assistance of a reputable sex counseling agency. (All of the foregoing,
women physicians will appreciate, reflects not a belief that all physicians are male but the deficit in our language of a sexless pronoun. The
choice between a male and a female physician as counselor to a particular patient of either sex often has to be made by trial and error, and
one may succeed where the other fails.)

For the doctor unwilling or unable to go beyond first-instance reassurance, referral is mandatory. Sexual problems, when they present,
often have gone on too long already, and they are aggravated by medical dickering. Referral to a sex clinic of teaching hospital quality is not
possible everywhere, even for paying patients. The psychiatrist will
certainly help where he can and is the referral of final or auxiliary
resort in all cases where major problems of identity are opened up or
the patient is mentally ill. Nevertheless, the psychiatrist's training is
not in the direct symptomatic types of intervention now being developed, and referral to him in the first place can reinforce the symptom
and enhance the patient's sense of abnormality. Behavioral therapy of
the modern, nonaversive, or reinforcing type—with or without biofeedback—is a possible referral and can be assessed for result or non-
result in the short term. But it is still confined to major centers.

One form of psychotherapy, or consciousness raising, that is almost
universally helpful to the sexually dysfunctional patient is peer group

discussion involving several couples with a trained, or at least a sexually experienced, leader couple. It is perhaps asking too much that a
group practice organize such a facility for its sexually dysfunctional
patients, but it can be done, using available tapes and literature and
the services of a consultant. Such physician leadership is immensely
valuable as an adjunct to more specific treatments. Remember that the
sexually dysfunctional or anxious person is badly imprisoned by privacy, regards his problems or peculiarities as both shameful and
unique, has difficulty in talking openly about them, and can be immensely relieved by the mere fact of hearing others do so. Problems of
body image, worthiness, sexual roles, and man-woman conflict—this
last a particularly sore point in our society—can be broached. Such a
group needs professional direction; do-it-yourself encounter in this
field can be destructive.

The reason for the ordinary physician to enter sex counseling—both
by experiencing and using it in office practice—is precisely that if he or
she does not, patients with sexual dysfunctions and associated identity
problems will seek do-it-yourself resources from which they may or
may not get comprehensive or judicious assistance. Becoming skilled,
compassionate sex counselors will involve hard work and goodwill,
but it seems clear that we should make the effort.

Sexuality In A Zero-Growth Society

A Verbatim Lecture

Throughout most of human history, marriage, even when it was monogamous, was not so much about sexual companionship as about kinship. By kinship I mean the movement of the individual across and within families, the acquisition of kin, and often the disposal of property. Women were not only sexual partners and potential mothers of descendants, but ambassadors between clans, and they were very often treated as walking bearer-bonds in that they brought inheritances with them; they gave access to the store of another family; or they had to be bought from their clan or their parents. One striking surviving instance of the dynastic use of women as access to the power of a clan is in the British legal provision that to ravish a queen or a princess who is heir to the throne is treason, not because it would be rough on the queen or the princess, but specifically to prevent usurpation by abduction, since the heir, even of a rape, would be entitled to royal pretensions.

The major change in this pattern, which is not really very far behind us in our thinking today, took place with the substitution of what is called the romantic idea of marriage. This was, roughly speaking, the ideology which affected to ignore dynastic and financial considerations (as some marriages always have done) and to substitute instead complete mutual absorption of the kind which one commonly sees among people who are in love. The change was that this "peak experience" was expected to be lifelong. The romantic concept was, I think, a psychological advance on the practical in many ways—it recognized the woman as a person and an equal chooser. It ran very well so long as the residue of the older kinship system and the relatively stratified society which it generated continued to be present. Its weaknesses were inherent, however, in the absence of an extended family and a local society, because the isolation which is sought by lovers can become a very burdensome experience for married people who are grossly overexposed to each other's society, and for children who are grossly overexposed to their parents. This sort of overexposure did not occur in the 19th century village where the community was much more open, but is very typical, I think, of the 20th century suburb. At the same time there were survivals still in our thinking of the old property basis of marriage, a basis in

117

which adultery really did involve a transaction a little like clipping coupons off somebody else's bearer-bond. This became transferred imperceptibly to the persons of spouses. It took the hard-headed Cockney to remark, as they always did among the working classes of London, "Nobody ever misses a slice off of a cake what's been cut." That was not the view of the middle classes. With the equalization which took place, both the husband and the wife ended up being owned by each other and the use of the term "cheating" which we still hear sometimes, implies that sort of ownership. So the unspoken consequence of this was that the husband might expect to exact total chastity from his wife, which he had very often done in the past, so as to know whose children were whose. The wife by way of compensation could enjoin on her husband what my wife once rather nicely called "penile servitude for life."

I think it is important to give this rather cynical view of the development of romantic marriage rather than one which portrays its advantages for personal development and mutual respect, over the dynastic structural kinship marriage which had gone before, because it is the caricature and not the fact which has determined the forces for further change, the misrepresentation and not the many satisfied customers. Anyone who doubts the validity of the caricature has only to look at the rubric of difficulty in marriage, namely the divorce laws of various countries.

Romantic marriage had several strengths—equality in choice, love rather than policy, and a higher valuation of the sexual. One found those things occasionally in an arranged marriage, and all were capable of providing either gains or problems. The weaknesses were the growing overexposure of the partners to each other with dwindling dilution by kin, friends, or society; the increase in personal dependency which went with that; the anxieties which were associated with the dependency; and the transfer of the property concept to persons. But other factors have arisen to destabilize the romantic-monogamous pattern, without which it might have proved satisfying to even more than the sizeable majority who still profess to accept it. One of these is the drastic reduction in early mortality. Far more Victorian marriages were terminated by death than modern marriages are terminated by divorce. Another is the advent of reliable control over conception. In a zero population growth society, the recreational and relational aspects of sex become much more important than its reproductive use. One important ethical and practical constraint—that children need a stable biparental setting in order to grow up undamaged—can be avoided by not having children. The shortage of kin which was already appearing early in the century as the huge Victorian family contracted, will become greater, and though kin can be a burden as well as a resource, they simply will not be available to dilute the mutual dependence of spouses.

Romantic marriage has reacted to these processes by a change of practice, most marked I think in Scandinavia and in America but reflected even in Catholic countries like Spain where religion reinforces the institution by dictating the public laws. The professed attitude, which our Japanese neighbors call the "front culture" as opposed to the back culture, is one of exclusive lifelong monogamy. I well remember a witness in court asking a judge, "What exactly do you mean by marriage?" The judge said, "Christian matrimony, Madam—Christian matrimony." The actual practice of a substantial proportion of couples is, in fact, serial polygamy. Marriages occur sequentially, since "marriage" is still required to disinfect intercourse. But they are ended more or less at will by divorce, and serial polygamy is also helped out by adultery. Couples resentful of the possessive ethic, as well they may be, or aware of the damage done by overexposure to a single partner, increasingly tolerate secondary relationships provided these are not "serious," are for sex only, do not overhumanize or value the third party and do not come too blatantly to the notice of the spouse or the neighbors. Adultery of this kind is not a new feature of monogamy; it was just as common as now in Chaucerian or in upperclass Victorian England—and is just as common today in Catholic countries where divorce is inadmissible. In the last of those it was institutionalized in the person of the mistress, the cavaliere servente, and what the Mexicans call "la casa chica"—the little house where you keep your mistress. In the modern scene, however, it has changed its role somewhat. We now feel uneasiness and dissatisfaction with yet another example of bad faith in the culture, with the idea that monogamy need in any event be an exclusive relationship emotionally, and with the idea that secondary relations can rightly be devalued or deprived of a humanness and openness which they could have. In all of these respects I think we are becoming more conscientious, not less moral.

Contemporary marriage is accordingly in a state of flux. It is a flux which was ably predicted many years ago by George Bernard Shaw in his pamphlet-play "Getting Married" in which he made every single point we are making here; a remarkable achievement if you consider when it was written. The worst sufferers from the confusion of earlier years were the children of serially married parents. Some of them underwent an experience which could be more disturbing than bereavement, the Victorian equivalent, and the acquisition of step-parents. Therefore, quite a few entrants to marriage now are the product of a disturbing growth experience within the family scene. I'm not thinking here in terms of disorders of imprinting but rather disorders of role, and also of a different valuation of roles, which need not necessarily be a disorder. Couples do still genuflect to the expectation of permanence. They start a family, but since divorce is available they resort to it as soon as the going gets tough.

A growing percentage of younger couples now appear to practice trial marriage. This is an old expedient in all rural cultures. We now use it to test compatibility. In 18th and 17th century England its use was to test the viability of the husband and wife team as farmers, because there was no use being married to somebody who couldn't make cheese and who couldn't do the other things that were necessary to make a farm profitable. Trial marriage, where you hired your wife at the fair for a year, was indeed an institution in late 17th and early 18th century England.

Expectation among educated people is apparently becoming more educated. Even the fantasy literature, on which we pattern ourselves, has moved away from the happy-ever-after themes which played a very large part in the miseducation of whole generations of young women. Literature is now getting to be rather more realistic about interpersonal relations. Society in general is moving away from the mutual-sufficiency, mutual-ownership stereotype (the couple who lock themselves up in a cottage with their own children, and are totally sufficient one unto another, who lay upon each other all of the expectations which should properly be laid on kin and society as well as on the spouse, and then are surprised when they quarrel). I think it is moving away from the pattern of two rival actor-managers trying to produce each other, which was a common fault of matrimony under the romantic dispensation. It's moving closer to the celebrated formulation of Fritz Perls, "I am I and you are you, and neither of us is here to live up to the other one's expectations, but when we meet it's beautiful."

Some legally recognized primary relationship seems to me quite insupplantable as the focus of man-woman relations in most cases, and there is absolutely no sign that the popularity of marriage is declining, in fact if anything, it is increasing. What I think is likely to happen is that it will become more open, that childbearing, by far the most important moral consequence of sexual activity, will be recognized both legally and by individuals as a chosen separate lifestyle which imposes limits on the freedom to dissolve a relationship; and that society will with this exception, move physical man-woman relations out of the conspicuous place which Christianity and convention have caused them to occupy in the field which we optimistically describe as "morals," and replace them with interpersonal and parental obligation—truly moral topics. Thus a far wider range of lifestyles will come to be accepted, and acceptable without any sort of guilt or obloquy—lifestyles will simply cease to be important topics of conversation or censure in society, even though many of those possible are always likely to be minority choices. Such variations have always existed under all marital systems—there have always been threesomes, there have always been spouse exchanges—people had to keep them under the rug for fear of what the neighbors would say. We shall approach the recognition of such behaviors without special note and with tolerance instead of that devastating anxiety, born of total dependency, which the old form of marriage generated. The demoralization of sex per se and the substitution of morals based on responsibility, especially to children, and on caring for people, represents a logical outgrowth of this striking change in the importance of the family. In Maslow's rather infelicitous phrase, we will tend to substitute "being-love" for "dependency love," and say with William Blake's Oothoon: "Can that be love that drinks another as a sponge drinks water?"

The ancient Jewish codes, still practiced by many Jews, which Christianity converted under its own proper motion into a quite extraordinary brand of antisexualism, really owed their logic originally to kinship considerations. Kinship was a foundation of all ancient law. Rational periods of Christian tradition and popular practice were also concerned with kinship; but with the idealization of celibacy in Catholic cultures and the fear of spontaneity and pleasure in Protestant Puritan cultures, all kinds of grotesque moralisms were grafted on. Such moralisms have nothing to do with the valid intuition that all sexual relations are potentially sacramental. Religious marriage meanwhile will obviously endure as long as does religion, which is probably as long as man, since all humans value rites de passage in matters which move them or concern them deeply.

It is possible that with the change in intellectual climate, and particularly with the shortage of kin, charismatic and Adamite religious and secular movements, which are already in evidence (though rarely now explicitly "religious"), and in which love and sexuality are universalized, may very well find a growing place. These are movements which systematize non-possession with love, an insight which monogamy has lacked: those who value possession as an index of love obviously find them threatening. They are very interesting to observe anthropologically because open sex experiences have a very disconcerting way of being far more religious in tone than they are lascivious. Open sex has an inherent quality of becoming a lay sacrament—very often to the surprise and the discomfiture of people who seek it in pursuit of "kicks" and who instead find innocence. It is a rather surprising outcome, but not surprising to an anthropologist who knows the uses of these behaviors in cultures other than our own. Nor would William Blake have found it surprising. The social use of sexuality, which seems to reflect a current trend in America today, also substitutes for the shortage of kin by the erotization of friendship, which is quite a new experience for our culture but fully traditional in others (such as the Eskimo where shortage of kin is truly a handicap: sexual exchange creates surrogate kin—you lent him your wife, you can borrow his canoe). Males in particular, both human and primate, who share a female are traditionally blood brothers, not rivals. While overt acceptance of such behaviors is now rather limited, the influence of ideas drawn from them, and stressing full equality and freedom with caring, is going to spread and is in fact already spreading. It is spreading to the solid middle class which has started fidgeting at its moorings when reading about open marriage, and which is beginning to accept the concept of the interchangeability, at least in nonreproductive marriage, of male and female roles which we find increasingly stressed by feminists. This applies both to work situations, and to the ethic in which women were formerly reared, which taught that feminine love can only be expressed in a total relationship. It was Byron who said that "Love is part of a man's life and all of a woman's." Most women now think that that notion is a canard, and their own self-experience shows the fact to be otherwise.

These are some of the changes which we are seeing already. If we examine today's society and today's sexual patterns, there are two fundamentally new factors we can identify. I have mentioned them both: one is the removal of specific sexual behaviors, which were the subject of nearly all of the moralistic prohibitive emphases of organized religion, from the control of a folklore created by a few disturbed people, and their translation into the field where they can be studied and observed. We have come to realize their prevalence and their lack of significance. We have come, for example, to recognize the basic normality, and the biological function and programming, of things such as masturbation and orogenitality, which have just come off the prohibited list. We are coming to recognize that humans are all potentially bisexual in being able under appropriate circumstances to respond erotically to stimuli from both sexes—though not all of them have sufficient pressure, whether educational, cultural, endocrine, or whatever, to respond in both ways. This whole revision of attitude amounts to the decriminalization of sex.

The other new factor is the direct consequence of reliable contraception which makes all the uses of sexuality separable. Human sexuality does not, and never did, exist primarily for reproduction in terms of numerical frequency. We mate all through pregnancy, we mate in the infertile parts of the month, and the majority of active couples mate at least every other day and sometimes much more frequently than that.

Accordingly, then, the biological functions of sexuality are three—reproductive certainly, relational secondarily, and recreational as well. In the past reproduction was a constant and inherent possibility, and largely because of it women were convinced by training that they could not worthily enjoy wholly recreational sex. Reproduction necessarily overshadowed every act of intercourse. Men were permitted, though not encouraged, to view sexuality not only as fatherhood but also as recreation, and the substance of much, much literature is the unhappy event where two people approached sexuality with differing views as to the universe of discourse: one of them thought of it as relationship and the other thought of it purely as recreation.

Sexual intercourse has also a fourth dimension, in effect, as an extended form of play—it is the most important form of adult play, worthy of a study as careful as that of Winnicott on the psychiatric uses of child play. It is quite clear that the exorcising of social and role anxieties is a perfectly proper function for sexual playfulness. In the case where some ritual or object is necessary for performance, that condition is almost a transitional object, like the teddy bear without which the child succumbs to anxiety. We do in fact see the classical pattern of displacement activities, both in child play and in the adult play implicit in sexual acting-out. In fact, any human act of intercourse can involve all of these or any combination of them, and this must be the first generation in much of Europe and the United States to accept recreational sex as socially worthy. It can do so because it can control pregnancy and doesn't any more have to divide women into mothers and wives who are good women, and playful people who are bad, a fantasy which contributed to a great deal of marital impotence in earlier days. Sex was not a nice thing to do to a nice girl. This notion still does contribute to the impotence we see in traditional-role males when confronted with a sexually positive woman.

Another valuable feature of "social" sex has been the opening of sexual behaviors to observation and comparison. Many individuals have had the opportunity of comparing partners. A high proportion of clinical sexual problems in the past have had their origin in privacy and in the fact that this is the only important skill which we don't normally learn by watching. We have the curious situation that generations of sex counselors were talking about behavior which they had never actually seen, except possibly in a mirror. And since sex on the couch described by an anxious patient to a psychiatrist or to a counselor differs quite radically in emphasis, in meaning, and in over-determinants from sex on the hoof, our whole medical view of normality was liable to distortion by our patients' anxieties. Ever since Krafft-Ebing, it's been the assignment of the physician and of the counseling community to go around converting all of the best turn-ons into hang-ups. That was the reaction of people who had had very little sex and who had observed none. The idea of Sigmund Freud actually watching sexual behavior is mindboggling.

Why are we insistent on sexual privacy? If you think about it, in order to analyze it, some people say, "This is a beautiful thing—we like to keep ourselves to ourselves." There is the "womb sense" which others express—of wishing to be alone with another person without any distraction. But another component of the desire for privacy implies that others are hostile, that what is being done is shame-producing because others will disapprove of it, they will interfere, they will call the police, they will steal our partner, or in some other way they will be unsupportive. In a supportive environment including other people, nonprivacy can have a very positive psychological impact, enhanced by its unconventionality.

Any move towards social uses of sexuality would have been impossible without a gradual change in attitude towards, and in anxiety about, bisexuality. Mate sharing, both psychoanalytically, and as we see it in primates, is a surrogate sexual relationship, usually between males in which the woman is a bridge (her traditional kin role, in fact). It is expressed covertly in our society in the "gang night out" and in the attraction of the prostitute as a shared woman because these are acceptable substitutes for any open male-male contact. This we taboo, and these are covert substitutes for it. It is my view that bisexuality is in fact a ground structure of human sexuality, but it is very hard to be certain of that, because society has walked all over it in its heaviest boots. We know very well that in ancient Greece it was a fashionable affectation to say, as Ovid did in Rome, "On the whole I like boys less than girls." Everybody who could assume that affectation did so even if it was not particularly to their taste.

In our society, a display of bisexual behavior, particularly by males, has been regarded as a disease or as a crime, and therefore only those displayed it who must. Therefore in overt behaviors, we see the extremes of the range: a wholly heterosexual norm and a homosexual abnorm. But a "homosexual" person is not one attracted by his or her own sex so much as one who finds difficulty in responding to the other sex. This concept now underlies much therapy, which aims to provide the dissatisfied homosexual with an additional option, not to suppress a preference. In fact, in a more open scene, normal women relate to each other physically without any inhibitions and without any indication that they are at all unable to relate to men. Men find it much harder to do that. In general, they will relate through the woman, though after a while they come to be a little more able on some occasions to relate to each other.

Both this surrogate pattern and the capacity for direct erotization of male-male relations seems to me probably adaptive in man. If we examine primates which have no such capacity, they tend to break up into hostile hordes in which the males are so jealous of each other that they don't form societies in which there is societal as well as family bonding. Gibbons are an example of this. The group is never bigger than the family tribe. In the past evolutionists have wondered how the human instability of sex object, and the human instability of sex role have survived. They look very disadaptive for breeding; it is surely the nadir of Darwinian unfitness to be fixated on an object like a pair of boots or a member of your own sex. I think the answer is that plasticity of object choice has probably had an adaptive function in evolution by making it possible for us to use sexuality for bonding, in the expression of dominance behaviors, and in many other social contexts accessible to indirect selection. I am also convinced that Maslow was right in thinking that dominance plays a very large part in the suppression of heterosexual drives, which is the real problem of people who are predominantly but unwillingly or anxiously homosexual. I think that in a fully erotized society bisexuality, whether it is expressed or not, will cease to be a problem about which a physician is consulted. We shall come to see it as a primate option, the expression of which has more to do with dominance than with heterosex gone wrong, and we'll be much less concerned about it. When Ovid wrote as he did, he wasn't very concerned about it.

Another important casualty in the process of change, I think, will be sexual jealousy. There's been an enormous amount of argument over how far jealousy is a normal emotion and the counterpart of love, and how far it is simply the product of propaganda (Othello was jealous because that was what was expected of him—he had no wish to strangle Desdemona, but it was the macho thing to do, so he did it). There's also the likelihood that jealousy which does not represent role-playing of this kind is merely the product of dependency. It was a nicely made point of Maslow, who classified love into being-love and dependency-love, that being-love is not jealous because it wants to give to the other person and dependency-love is bound to be jealous because it fears losing the other person, an inevitable event in a mortal organism. There are two reactions to seeing "your person" displaying sexual affection for somebody else. One is to say, "He or she is extremely desirable and I love him or her, so obviously other people will like him or her too and I feel reinforced by it." The other reaction is the one prescribed by society and by anxiety, which requires that we act like a backward five year old who sees another child with his tricycle. After all the tricycle isn't going to be spoiled by being ridden. It would probably be true to say that in the traditional old-time family, jealousy was based on reproduction—the point was "knowing my children are mine." The great discovery of early man was not that sex produced babies—he discovered that early on—but that one act of sex produced babies, so that it was possible to establish who was whose father. Before that there was no argument who was whose mother, but once fathers got the chance of staking a claim, they began to do so.

In romantic couple situations jealousy is a product of the fear of rejection which comes from a surrender which is so alarmingly total. This pattern may have expressed revolt against the need to share affection with numerous siblings. That belonged to a past generation—it will be interesting to see if the children of one-child families are more or less able or needing to display jealousy when they reach the marriageable age. I know of no work on that. Modern attempts to transcend jealousy through open sex and ritualized wife exchange, through greater tolerance of affairs, and by a general revision of attitude to mutual ownership are uncertain and anxious, but also involve acceptance of a more realistic view of the couple, of the individual's needs and of the difference between primary and subsidiary relationships. Above all they contain the recognition that if you love somebody, meeting their needs rather than frustrating them seems to be the natural way to behave, and an approach which in practice strengthens the primary bond. One doesn't need to copy the mischief-making lovers of "Les Liaisons Dangereuses" to recognize this. A revision of the prescription of jealousy as a "good" attitude will be a very important change if it comes about, because it will mark the end of the mutual proprietorship which has so often characterized human sexual relations in the past. I think that our grandchildren may find it very hard to understand what 19th century opera, with all of its jealousies and uproar about who sleeps with whom, is about.

In brief then, contraception has given us control over our reproduction and has made it possible to separate the human uses of sexuality.

Ethological study of the variety of sexual behaviors has decriminalized sex and taken it out of the sphere of irrational fear and shame. The combination of these changes, coming into a society in which few older models of kinship are active, has given us a new valuation, or at least a revival of a primitive valuation not previously seen in a developed society—that sex is not only a matter of couple-binding, but also a form of social intercourse, an erotized version of friendship, largely recreational, partly relational, sometimes charismatic in a religious manner, and only reproductive by choice: it is what one does with close friends. In fact, the only further discovery needed to make that virtually general is to remove the last of "God's little allies," as they've been called, and to give us an esthetic genital antiseptic. All of these are old anthropological uses of sexuality, but what has made them newly available is the reliable control of reproduction.

Most people's behaviors remain traditional, but the trend does seem to me unmistakable. Nobody writing a sociosexual scenario for the 2000's could ever exclude wild cards—for example, a Billy Graham-type revival of reproductivism, of a babies-are-beautiful, back-to-the-family, God-meant-us-to-breed social philosophy. If that became a cult it could turn demographic trends around literally overnight. It only takes a very few minutes to produce a baby and if everybody does it, you are going to have a great number of babies.

We have to go with the most likely prevision and that seems to be as follows: there obviously will be no abandonment of marriage, and I think people who have predicted it are wrong. That is to say, marriage as a two-person legal arrangement will become much more stable, for two reasons:

1) We will have taken sexual exclusivity out of the picture so people will cease to be quarreling about who sleeps with whom—they will regard marriage as a much more stable and social relationship, just as the traditional kinship marriage largely ignored adultery which wasn't public. Sexual relations will have become a social gesture—something which occurs between friends and will therefore tend to stabilize primary relationships by removing the denial element and the exclusivity from them.

2) Parenthood will become a distinct and nonaccidental lifestyle, and I think it will be maintained in that form by very strong, science-based social pressures. What the form will have to be will depend on further research on what it is that disorganizes development in childhood. But, to take an example, in the past if two men and a woman had announced they would set up house and had made it clear they intended all three of them to engage in sexual relations with each other, they would have incurred very powerful disapproval from a lot of social, a lot of legal, and possibly even criminal sanctions. Society was applying a very strong pressure against that type of behavior. I think future societies will regard that sort of idiosyncratic choice as morally quite unimportant—most people will say, "Sooner them than me." But the same social and legal disapproval and pressure will be reserved for people who bear children they don't want, who neglect or abuse children they have, who create serial families, who fail to treat the reproductive use of sex with the moral seriousness it requires. Morals will have been displaced from the external genitalia where they have very little place into the uterus where they properly belong. When you remember that in several states every year there are a number of cases of divorce in which neither party wants custody of the children, you begin to see the sort of behavior which our descendants will, I hope, view censoriously. It won't be the things about which the past was censorious. And one would hope that other things about which they'll be censorious and shocked will be exploitive and selfish non-reproductive sexual behaviors of all kinds, so that not only moral obloquy but "good manners" will be mobilized to produce community pressure against them. There's no more powerful pressure. Nobody minds being thought a devil, but every boy hates to be thought an ill-mannered boor.

Physicians have seldom taken up these issues occupationally and explicitly. Physicians reading this may wonder why I'm discussing such topics and where they stand in this changing scene. The answer is, I think, on the sidelines—making your own personal choices of behaviors, as all citizens must do, but not attempting, as in the past, to function as custodians and censors of the choices your patients make. It's quite important that we recognize this because we have an obligation in counseling. Physicians need, without sacrificing the traditional professional ethic of not having sex with their patients (which is a very good one, needs to be maintained and is going to be harder to maintain if social sex becomes increasingly conventional), to understand the stresses of a change in society as profound as that which we are now undergoing, and they need to qualify themselves by getting abreast of modern counseling. Magic sex, which is what we had in the past, carried with it a heavy burden of guilt. Private sex has a big burden of performance anxiety; and it's the allaying of anxieties which has been the biggest quantitative assignment of sexual counseling. You may remember the formula—it starts by giving permission, then limited information, then special information, and only if those fail do you need to resort to treatment. A more open sexual scene, with its opportunities to observe the performance of others,

immediately creates other anxieties in the form of competition and rejection fears—the sort of fears we all experienced in adolescence. We
already see people who are anxious, not as to whether it is ladylike for
a woman to move, or whether it is sinful for a woman to enjoy, but
people who wonder why the orgasm they are having is not as big as
the one they can hear coming through the wall from next door. It's no
use explaining that just as some people scream with laughter, others
do not, and that humans are demonstrative in ways that depend on
culture and individuality; the fear persists.

The creation of anxiety is a human tendency and we are going to
have a job to mitigate it by the exposure of games-playing and by
doing all we can to create what Sartre used to call "good faith." I don't
think that means going back to that terrible over-seriousnes of the old
Judaeo-Christian tradition where sex was never fun. One function of
non-reproductive sex is playfulness. The seriousness belongs to relationship and it belongs to childbearing—it does not belong to sexuality.
Even then we don't need to produce guilty and anxious parents by
suggesting to them, as was suggested to the parents of many autistic
children, that it was their own fault because of rejection, when the
condition was almost certainly organic in origin. I think there are psychoanalytic grounds for thinking that we shall not as a culture come to
terms with generous human sexuality until we are ready to come to
terms with death, which is the last enemy of love. Death is the ultimate
generator of "good faith" and nontriviality. If you want to see the real
valuation of sexuality in relationship, you want to hear it discussed in
a group therapy session of terminal patients. You'll hear more "good
faith" there than you will in most discussions that take place before
we confront eternity.

I think we shall see a movement towards the situation Devereux described in the South Sea Islanders—a very different one from our own.
We have been taught to believe that sex is what you do with people
you love. The South Sea Islanders have been taught to believe love is
what you get from people with whom you have good sex. I think it is
possible for both of these interactions to exist, but that we shouldn't
reject one or the other provided the contacts are genuine, innocent and
caring. We, as physicians, are not in business to promote any particular ethos for the structure of human relations. I think we are on the
verge of a period in which family primary-care medicine is coming
back with an improved version of the traditional social commitment of
the physician *as* a physician, not as a tradesman, or as a technician, or
as something other than a physician. In that setting, if that is so, we are
going to need to look forward to the kind of family we shall be dealing
with, both the reproductive and the non-reproductive, the conven-

130

tional and the unconventional, so that whatever kind of house we enter, we do so in order to heal. We cannot avoid the possession of attitudes, nor should we—but we need to be aware of them in ourselves. It's what you *signal* to your patient, not what you say to him. If you can't avoid displaying judgmental attitudes that alarm or cause general discomfiture, you'd better stay off the subject.

The valuation of sexual experience is changing, and a large part of our counseling function as physicians-counselors will lie in this area if we are willing to prepare ourselves for it. We are part of society and if it changes we shall have to change. You may know that research on medical school entrants some years ago showed that they were then the group with the most sexual problems of entrants to any profession. One could, if one wanted to, invent psychoanalytic reasons for this assertion. But as medicine moves with the general flow of society, it is a state we must remedy both by medical education and by personal growth.

IV
On Gerontology
Geriatrics—
The Missing Discipline

Demography and our own experience tell us that the medicine of the last quarter of the lifespan—geriatrics—will be the major component in future office practice; all the more so since, along with a rise to between 12 and 14 in the overall percentage of citizens over 65 by the end of the century, goes the fact that the characteristic pathology of aging is an increase in the number of pathologies. Older people need more doctor hours.

The word *geriatrics* was invented in the U.S. by Nascher, and it is one of the astonishments of the European immigrant doctor that in the land of medical technology, geriatrics as Europeans know it hardly exists. Outside of a few great Jewish hospitals and a few exemplary sites, it is not taught as an obligatory discipline and is regarded as something that the competent internist does not need to learn. In Europe it was long since learned from the pioneer work of men like Ferguson Anderson that the incurable, incontinent, demented, image of old age is a social artefact, that its appearance clinically is as often as not iatrogenic, and that old people can be treated and cured whenever the same condition in a younger person can be treated and cured.

A medicine without geriatrics looks to Europeans as lopsided as a medicine without pediatrics. The diseases, symptomatology and therapeutics of babies differ from those of vigorous adults. So do those of the old. Pneumonia which induces convulsions in an infant and delirium in an adult can present in the old person with only one symptom—confusion—and only one immediate sign—an increase in respiratory rate. Other signs are of course present, but a physician who believes, as many once did, that mental confusion requires no explanation beyond chronological age may not look for them. The heart attacks of the old can be painless and present as sudden mental deterioration. The response of the old to drugs can be anomalous. The commonest causes of mental impairment at high ages are medication and physical disease, not chronic brain syndrome. There is no mystique about geriatrics, nor should it become, beyond a limited extent, a specialism. It simply needs to be learned, and at present the U.S. offers few opportunities and no obligation for the graduate to acquire it. With the probable advent of comprehensive health care, senior citizens will become an increasing part of the caseload: the country will suddenly realize that it lacks geriatricians, and after a period of private enterprise leading to public outcry, it will start importing them from Europe, with serious repercussions on the health care delivery to old people in Scandinavia, Britain, Canada and Holland, where geriatrics have advanced the furthest.

Confusion of this kind can be avoided and the need for older Americans to share access to the kind of quality geriatrics which their neighbors enjoy can be met if we start creating cadres now. This could best be done by exchange fellowships with European and Canadian geriatricians. In the meantime, while we prepare to teach all students, the practitioner who wants to keep up with this field can easily do so from the literature: Brocklehurst's "Textbook of Geriatric Medicine" is an excellent reference work. The aim of geriatric evangelism in America is not to create specialists beyond a few University chairs to match the 14 full professorships of geriatric medicine in Britain: in British and European experience, the best deliverer of geriatric care is the family practitioner.

Old people lack mobility when sick and require house calls. When sick, too, they often suffer from several distinct pathologies, which cannot be treated simultaneously without overprescribing. They thus present a notable test of therapeutic skill in assessing priorities, and their medication requires the constant supervision which only the family practitioner can give. They offer a constant challenge to the physician—it is much simpler to diagnose a diazepam deficiency or repeat a multiple prescription—and require that he operate in the context of a longterm awareness of the natural history of the patient and his environment which only the family practitioner readily acquires. Beside scientific medicine, the old person requires counsel, both as he or she enters old age with the negative mythology drawn from the culture, and in forecasting future changes such as lack of mobility or loss of the ability to drive, which need forward planning with the physician's assistance. The psychiatry of old age involves support—often against other family members who vent their problems on the old—and expertise in recognizing the physical causation of mental impairment, which may be cured by the simple discontinuance of some long-taken pharmacological prop, once tolerated but now producing side effects. In prescribing, the enemies of the older person are over-sedation, failure to diagnose and treat depression, and drugs which disorder electrolyte balance, cause dizziness or postural hypotension, or—simply—are multiple.

Geriatrics, accordingly, is a field for the physician who enjoys the practice of really testing medicine in every field. It cannot be auto-mated or conducted on a conveyor-belt principle, and it requires time. In Britain, the incentive to study it is provided by the payment of a higher annual capitation fee for every patient over 65 on the family practitioners' lists, plus an added payment in respect of acquiring credit in geriatrics. The British health care system has done much to promote this type of expertise; it resembles American democracy in that while citizens constantly criticize it, only the insane would wish to do away with it. Its emphasis on the role of family practice appeals to those who welcome the opportunity to be physicians in the to-tal sense; such men make good geriatricians for the reasons I have stated. The United States has yet to work out a system of health care delivery, but when this takes place, the availability of the geriatrician-family practitioner will be crucial to its success, whatever its fiscal or administrative form.

In the meantime the acquisition of geriatric training other than by reading is difficult; seminars, when these are held, are usually well at-tended. It should be a task of family medicine to increase the number of opportunities which we have to acquire new knowledge in this area—the knowledge exists and is constantly growing, the only prob-lem being the lack of exchange with pioneer European centers. In the growth of British geriatrics among family doctors, not only medical schools but the Royal College of Physicians and the Royal Society of Medicine did much to organize credit courses, case conferences and other means for the exchange of experience. It would be my hope that the American institutions concerned with postgraduate medicine will address themselves to geriatrics with equal success. In dealing with our most numerous patients we can use any information we can get.

The Myth of Senility

In view of the prevalence of genetic diseases apparent in infancy, and the rarity of those first appearing in old age, unexplained ill health is far more commonly idiopathic in pediatric than in geriatric practice. The attitude of prescientific medicine to the major infectious diseases of infancy in some respects resembled the attitude which considers senility as a diagnosis, in that it attributed to age (in this case, infancy) phenomena which in adults would be recognized as specific pathologies. In the case of the old, these are specific pathologies in which the signs and symptoms of textbook medicine, which is predominantly the medicine of adult and middle life, are muted or altered by aging and obscured by the persisting misconception that disability can be attributed to chronologic age alone.

Old people do not, in fact, become weak, frail, immobile, or demented through any common or near-universal change coupled to chronologic age in the way that loss of hair pigment is coupled. Their liability to pathologies, particularly multiple pathologies, increases, and although a high proportion of persons over age 65 describe themselves as being well, about 80 per cent suffer from one or more chronic conditions, which may be minor in their impact on function; and the 10 to 15 per cent who are seriously unwell commonly have more than one such condition. In these evidently ill patients, senility is no more than a slightly derogatory term for the physical and mental concomitants of chronic and explainable ill health.

When senility presents alone, and in the absence of any history of ill health, it means an ongoing loss of function from an occult cause which in a younger person would lead to intensive investigation, but in the old is treated as something to be expected. The main achievement of geriatric medicine, and the main requirement for its effective practice on the European model, is the liquidation of this erroneous belief.

Senility is not a complaint of the patient but a report by an old person's relatives or custodians. The patient may complain of weakness, loss of activity, or confusion, and attribute these changes to age. In either event, the factual basis is that there is a change so that the patient can no longer do what he or she recently did. In popular use, seni'ity refers to the loss of intellectual function or even to resentful or inconvenient behavior which, however justified by the setting, can be charitably attributed to such loss. The following case is a good example of how senility presents in clinical practice.

> The father of a distinguished geriatrician was an active and feisty man in his mid-80s, twice a widower, and a wayward pursuer of his own concerns. His son was notified by an alarmed family that "Dad is failing": he sat in a chair, and no longer showed an interest in women or in food. More seriously, he had three times forgotten where he had parked his car, and had reported it stolen. On the first two occasions, the police were tolerant—on the third, they suggested that the patient might have outlived his eligibility for a driver's license. A local practitioner diagnosed "old age." On examination, the patient was rational but a little confused, and the fire had gone out of him. He was also losing weight and experiencing fatigue on moving about.

I will return to this case later, because the outcome is instructive. The patient was fortunate, in America, in having a geriatrician in the family—in less affluent or less supportive circumstances he would have risked admission to a custodial institution, sedation in response to his anger at the procedure, and early death from medical neglect or the civilized equivalent of black magic. This is a not uncommon outcome of symptomatic disorientation in the old when senility is treated as a diagnosis—the Shakespearian last act.

While this popular reading of senility covers the actual symptoms of confusion and memory loss, hostile or difficult behavior, and dementia, which point to wholly different probable causes, equally common modes of presentation are weakness and loss of mobility in the absence of obvious cause such as arthritic pain (often described as "getting frail" or "going off his feet"), fatigue, and a general lack of appetency, including anorexia, loss of interest in events, and "giving up on life." Again, these symptoms are often charitably interpreted by relatives as a fitting and even natural preparation for the cue to "leave the stage."

Often the onset of this downward slope in the life of the patient is presaged by a series of unexplained falls, known as "premonitory falls" in geriatric parlance. These may represent not only neurologic disorders such as unrecognized parkinsonism or ingravescent stroke, but one of the common presentations in the elderly of heart attack, heart failure, chest or urinary infection, or the equally ingravescent side effects of medication.

The common thread in all of these senile manifestations is that *in old age the presentation of major illness is commonly nonspecific.*

Moreover, the popular reading of senility as "second childishness" cannot be separated from the physical pathologies which occur in age, because confusion, memory loss, and behavioral and mood changes are increasingly often symptomatic of major illness in older patients, as delirium is symptomatic of febrile illness in the young—the difference being that these may be the only symptoms in the elderly.

The commonest psychiatric disorders of old age are not senile dementia (organic and structural loss of brain function) and arteriosclerotic dementia (the sum of successive small infarctions rather than a decline in blood supply to the brain), but symptomatic clouding of consciousness and endogenous depression, with approximately equal frequency. Endogenous depression in the old may present as hypochondria or pseudodementia, be accompanied by loss of activity and interest, and rapidly impair physical health. It is also treatable by appropriate antidepressant therapy.

Symptomatic confusion, memory loss, or agitation can result from any silent infection, cerebrovascular or coronary occlusion, electrolyte disturbance from any cause, and the effects of medication. In contrast to the major organic dementias, these symptomatic changes are often (though not always) less gradual in onset, and they are transient if the cause is removed before grave physical and social damage has been done. The major disease process may differ from its typical adult form in being painless (coronary occlusion), afebrile (pneumonia, pyelitis), and attended by minimal signs.

Symptomatic mental illness in the old, whether it presents as memory loss, acute confusion, or apathy, is usually recognized when it occurs in the presence of obvious sickness. Unfortunately, this is often not the case. Mental symptoms of what is in fact minor delirium presenting as the only evidence of disorder can be the first or sole evidence of pneumonia, urinary infection, uremia, congestive heart failure, minor cerebral infarction without other gross neurologic signs, diabetic ketosis or hypoglycemia, and hypothermia. Old persons living in cold areas and inadequate housing are especially prone to hypothermia; this condition appears to be commoner, or more recognized, in Europe.

In all of these cases, the myth of senility may lead the incautious physician to miss the underlying pathology—a serious matter, because where this is treatable, mental function usually recovers completely. So long as the mental association between age and dementia persists, the minimal increase in respiratory rate of afebrile pneumonia or the presence of urinary infection can be missed. The prescribing of minor sedatives and other injudicious interventions directed to quiet the "demented" patient can add to the mischief. Institutionalization in a custodial "home" is in itself a potent cause of nocturnal confusion, especially in the already sick; and the treatment of this with chemical restraint constitutes an unintentional form of euthanasia in a patient whose mental confusion could be cured if minimal efforts at diagnosis were made.

Medication as a causative factor

Next to infection, the commonest cause of senility presenting with confusion is medication. For this reason, the first step taken in its investigation by European geriatricians is the plastic bag test, the assembling in one bag of all the substances—prescribed, bought, and borrowed—which the patient has been ingesting. These may number several dozen, and rarely number less than five or six. The second step is the cessation of all such medication which is not life-sustaining. Let us go back to the case which I cited before.

The geriatrician's father received a careful physical examination which showed no sign of infection or any other of the common physical causes of his condition. He denied taking any medication. Diligent inquiry, however, revealed that at the death of his first wife, many years before, he had been unable to sleep. Since that time, he had taken a single butabarbital tablet every night. When his second wife died, five years ago, he again could not sleep, and added a single nightly Quaalude tablet. This trifling amount of medication was stopped, despite his protests. Within ten days, the patient's activity and appetency returned. He ate well, pursued comely women, and never again mislaid his car. The patient's strength and posture also greatly improved with reversal of mild osteomalacia that had resulted from the microsomal-inductive effect of the barbiturate.[1]

The meaning of weakness and memory loss

Physical strength, in athletic terms, normally declines with age, but because such a decline is also normally gradual, the patient adjusts to it. Weakness of rapid onset, similar to that experienced in earlier life after a severe illness, is always symptomatic. It may conceal increasing dyspnea, or clinically predictable conditions such as anemia, but in the old, other less familiar causes such as spontaneous or drug-induced osteomalacia ("senile" rickets) may operate.

Another cause of weakness is the myopathy of silent hyperthyroidism. Excessive secretion of T_3 and T_4 can occur in the aged with or without exophthalmos, restlessness, and thyroid enlargement; in the "apathetic" form of thyrotoxicosis, weakness may be severe enough to inhibit even leisurely movement. Bahemuka and Hodkinson[2] found an incidence of 2.2 per cent unrecognized hypothyroidism and over 1 per cent unrecognized hyperthyroidism in aged subjects, both presenting with the nonspecific syndrome of "failure to thrive."

Both weakness and confusion can result from heart failure, either following a painless coronary episode or as the convergence on an aging myocardium of several trivial stresses which can combine to induce decompensation.[3] Weakness alone characterizes the sodium depletion of the syndrome of inappropriate antidiuretic hormone secretion (SIADH), which can complicate or be the presenting symptom of infection, malignancy, and myxedema.[4] Sodium depletion is also readily induced by the officious use of diuretics—one of the commonest medications used by the old.

Weakness can also mask the stiffness of parkinsonism, which can occur without evident tremor but responds to L-dopa therapy. Hodkinson[1] emphasized the importance of Wartenberg's head-drop sign[5] as a test for rigidity.

The treatment of hypertension in the old, if based on criteria appropriate for a younger patient, can induce a form of senility ranging from weakness due to hypokalemia or hyponatremia to loss of confidence from postural hypotension, lowering of mood caused by ganglion blocking agents, and interference with sexual function from the same cause.[6] These side effects of many antihypertensive therapies can render the cure more onerous than the disease at earlier ages, but their effects are particularly prominent in the old, where treatment of nominal hypertension can severely disorder both well-being and brain function.

In common with other responses, recall becomes slower with age. This effect, which troubled Thomas Jefferson and led him to argue against a life presidency, is most prominent in those least mentally active, but causes the most anxiety to the intellectual. It is benign and nonprogressive, however. Severe deterioration of memory can herald the major dementias, but equally common or commoner causes are undiagnosed myxedema and hangover due to the use, even in normally acceptable doses, of any sedative drug. There are no "minor tranquilizers" in geriatrics, nor should the normal later-life pattern of light sleep and frequent waking be medicated. This needs to be distinguished from the early waking characteristic of depressive illness, however.

It is important to recognize that behavior which is odd in the young is interpreted as senility in the old, by common consent of the culture. The young man who assaults little girls is seen as psychopathic; the old man who does so, even when his access to more normal sexual gratification is restricted by opportunity or by infirmity, is described as senile.

Persons whose behavior was odd in youth may become odder with age as the pressure of societal rejection comes to bear on them. Paranoia, at any age, is a cover for unexplainable experiences. In the old, it may be an attempt to cover sensory losses such as deafness, cortical blindness, or symptomatic amnesias. It may also express the psychic recognition of the hostility of relatives. Anomic behavior and self-neglect can represent a gradual increase in confusion and weakness from remediable or irremediable causes. Sometimes this loss of ability to tend oneself is compounded by personal pride which makes the patient unwilling to let others see him or her in a neglected condition.

The idea that old people are more commonly lonely than the young, except after bereavement, may well be exaggerated as a cause of depression. Where isolation and depression coexist in the old, the isolation and neglect are quite commonly results of endogenous depression rather than causes of reactive depression.

Senility and loss of morale

Loss of morale is inherent in the concept of senility itself. At all other ages and in all other conditions, society, while it may not be supportive of disability, tends to support the attempt of the patient to cope. In the aged, the pressure is in the other direction—to accept the fitness, propriety, and naturalness of decline, and to bury prematurely the older person, fit or ailing, by a process of social devaluation. Hardy individuals in reasonable health can resist this pressure, but the symptoms I have described tend to excite in the elderly invalid, however robust his or her self-image, the anxiety that society may be right after all. It is in age that we most often see the syndrome of self-willed death[1,7] otherwise confined to those who believe in the efficacy of sorcery. One function of the geriatrician is accordingly as a breaker of spells cast by the folklore of old age.

Investigation of senility

The investigation of senility resolves itself into the careful search for the underlying pathology, the removal of iatrogenic disease where present, and the healing in patients, relatives, and physicians themselves of the sorcery wrought by the assumption of causeless infirmity as a feature of old age.

The minimal exclusionary approach to senility involves a proper history; a full physical examination carried out with patience (no simple matter where confusion or deafness limits cooperation), with special attention to infections and to the signs, often minimal, of endocrine and metabolic disorders; and a battery of tests directed to the known causes of nonspecific illness. For such a battery, Hodkinson[1] suggests an x-ray examination of the chest with attention to signs of infection, pulmonary edema, neoplasm, and bony changes, including fractures and Looser's lines in the scapula; blood cell count (Coulter Counter, Model S); measurement of BUN and electrolytes, serum albumin and globulin, and alkaline phosphatase; blood sugar (random sample); T_3 and T_4 uptake; and routine urinalysis.

To these should be added a thorough inquiry into and reevaluation of *all* medications. This should be carried out with reference to a geriatric textbook, not the manufacturer's literature, since the list of precautions and side effects required by the FDA contains no special reference to drug hazards in the aged. All medication not evidently life-sustaining may well be withdrawn, with due attention to possible effects of sudden discontinuance and to the interaction of retained and withdrawn drugs, e.g., through loss of ribosomal induction.

When the investigation is complete, and symptoms have remitted or have been explained, only those medications which are clearly indicated should be reinstated. These should not exceed four or five, however numerous the pathologies identified. Sedatives, antihypertensives, and diuretics are the most abused drugs in older persons. They are rarely or never indicated for prolonged use.

In view of the commonness of confusion as a symptom in the old, it is wise to test specifically for orientation and memory as part of the standard physical examination. On the other hand, elderly patients in full possession of their faculties need not be affronted and alarmed on admission by abrupt enquiries whether they know what year it is and who is President.

Most of the standard test material can be included in history taking. A patient who knows the answers to unthreatening and natural questions such as his or her name, address, date of birth, name of next of kin, and time and place of appointment is unlikely to be severely disoriented. Five-minute recall of an address given at the end of the history taking should be openly tested. Counting backward from 20, an important test of control over mentation, should be specifically included in examination of the central nervous system. In this way, no information is lost, and the confidence and dignity of an already apprehensive patient are not clumsily injured to the detriment of future communication.

In the presence of mental changes in the old, the essential task is to distinguish between symptomatic confusion, psychosis, and true dementia. The gradual onset of degenerative brain syndrome and the step-wise ingravescence of atherosclerotic (infarctive) dementia are characteristic where they occur, but symptomatic confusion can also be chronic or episodic. Goldfarb developed a mental status questionnaire,[8] and stressed its use in conjunction with Bender's double simultaneous stimulation (face-hand) test in detecting pseudodementia.[9] Psychometric tests, however, cannot always discriminate reversible from irreversible mischief, and the proper approach is exclusionary, since even in the presence of some organic impairment, intercurrent illness can produce reversible exacerbation and make the difference between impaired performance and frank dementia.

Of the typical psychoses, depression is the commonest and the most commonly overlooked. It can coexist with or simulate organic brain damage. Depression should be suspected and a therapeutic test made wherever mental dulling in the aged is accompanied by early waking, anorexia, and inert or miserable behavior and ideas.

Mania, because it is commonly hostile rather than expansive in the aged, is readily labeled senility and punished by sedation rather than treated. Lithium has been shown to be effective therapy for mania in the old as well as the young.[10]

When all psychiatric skills have been exhausted and all other causes of mental impairment excluded, there remain the major dementias—infarctive or of the Alzheimer type. Intensive work has produced a variety of drugs for their palliation,[11,12] but the true hope for the control of these conditions lies in the recognition that they are possibly viral or autoimmune diseases[13] or chemically expressed abiotrophies with a genetic component,[14,15] resembling, in this respect, Huntington's chorea.

The major dementias are common in age as measles is common in childhood, but their relation to chronology has no greater inevitability than that. They now fall within the rubric of investigable and preventable disease from which the culture-based notion of senility has so long excluded them, as it has excluded the old from the support of society and from the interest and engagement of the active physician.

Cases referred to a geriatric psychiatry unit are of three kinds—missed instances of symptomatic mental impairment due to identifiable illness or drugs; cases of newly appearing dementia or psychosis for expert consultation and diagnosis; and cases having some psychiatric feature and otherwise uninteresting to the general physician, which by reason of the patient's age can be unloaded on the geriatrician.

Prevalence of the first type of case will depend on the standard of geriatric diagnosis in primary care—they are commoner in the U.S. than in Britain, but occur in both countries. Cases of the second kind are clearly proper referrals. Cases of the third kind include the patient with longstanding parkinsonism in whom dementia or hallucinations develop, either from the disease or as a side effect, and the patient with residual cerebral damage from any cause who wanders, is aggressive, or is otherwise difficult to manage. This material, though unpromising in the eyes of those who refer the patients, is an important area for research. A geriatric unit can develop the expertise in medication needed to make life as bearable as possible for those who reach old age irremediably sick, and for their relatives.

More than patients of any other age, however, senile patients who do not respond to an exclusionary search for simple causes illustrate the confluence of pathology, age, and life situation. A typical example of this is the patient with longstanding personality problems who has had a stroke and shows intellectual impairment, who has suffered the loss of a spouse, who can no longer cope with his or her family situation, whose money has run out, and whose life-support systems have collapsed. Disease, the backlog of problems previously in equilibrium, bereavement, the social devaluation of the old in our culture, and poverty tend to strike together.

Physician, psychiatrist, neuropharmacologist, and social worker cannot "cure" these cases, though they can alleviate and, sometimes, heal. If such a collusion of misfortune occurred in younger adults it would be a focus of sympathy and of intensive research. Good geriatrics and better social attitudes may bring similar support to the old.

References

1. Hodkinson, H.M.: Common Symptoms of Disease in the Elderly. Oxford, England, Blackwell Scientific Publications, 1976.

2. Bahemuka, M., Hodkinson, H.M.: Screening for hypothyroidism in elderly inpatients. Brit. Med. J. 2:601-603, 1975.

3. Pomerance, A.: Cardiac pathology in the aged. Mod. Geriatrics 2:140-145, 1972.

4. Bartter, F., Schwartz, W.B.: The syndrome of inappropriate secretion of antidiuretic hormone. Am. J. Med. 49:790-806, 1967.

5. Wartenberg, R.: Head-dropping test. Brit. Med. J. 1:687-689, 1952.

6. Jackson, G., Pierscianowski, T.A., Mahon, W., et al.: Inappropriate antihypertensive therapy in the elderly. Lancet 2:1317-1318, 1976.

7. Milton, G.W.: Self-willed death, or the bone-pointing syndrome. Lancet 1:1435-1436, 1973.

8. Kahn, R.L., Pollack, M., Goldfarb, A.I.: Factors relative to individual differences in mental states of the institutionalized aged. In Hoch, P.H., Zubin, J.: Psychopathology of Aging. New York, Grune & Stratton, 1961.

9. Goldfarb, A.I.: Geropsychiatry in the general hospital. Mt. Sinai J. Med. N.Y. 38:79-88, 1971.

10. Foster, J.R., Gershell, W.J., Goldfarb, A.I.: Lithium treatment in the elderly. I. Clinical usage. J. Gerontol. 32:299-302, 1977.

11. Sathanathan, G.L., Gershon, S.: Cerebral vasodilators: A review. *In* Gershon, S., Raskin, A.: Genesis and Treatment of Psychological Disorders in the Elderly: Aging. Vol. 2. New York, Raven Press, 1975, pp. 155-168.

12. Lehmann, H.L., Ban, T.A.: CNS stimulants and anabolic substances in geriatric therapy. *In* Gershon, Raskin,[11] pp. 179-202.

13. Gajdusek, D.C.: Slow and latent viruses in the aging nervous system. *In* Maletta, G.: Survey Report on the Aging Nervous System. DHEW (NIH) Publication No. 74-296. Washington, DC, US Government Printing Office, 1974, pp. 149-168.

14. Davison, A.N.: Chemical pathology of brain degeneration. Proc. Roy. Soc. Med. 70:349-350, 1977.

15. Heston, L.L., Mastri, A.R.: The genetics of Alzheimer's disease: Associations with hematologic malignancy and Down's syndrome. Arch. Gen. Psychiat. 34:976-981, 1977.

Alzheimer's Disease or "Alzheimerism"?

With changes in demography and the introduction of phenothiazines, chronic brain syndromes are coming to occupy the place filled in the 19th century by neurosyphilis as the prime institutionalized mental disorder. Epidemiological and preventive research now focuses on two forms of this condition—the vascular-embolic and the primary or atrophic. While the first of these is an obvious target for prevention, along with hypertension, vascular disease, and embolic phenomena in other organs, the second has been studied with far less optimism because of the belief that it represented a statistically frequent part of a normal aging process. This belief, which reflects in part the folkloristic attitude to age as a source of mental incapacity—Shakespeare's "last act"—is now open to serious question; and "senile dementia" is being seen as a major epidemic disease which, like "general paralysis of the insane" (once regarded with similar fatalism), is comprehensible and probably preventable. Like other major CNS disorders which increase in frequency with age it shows genetic association, is accompanied by structural and immunologic changes, selectively affects certain brain areas and neurochemical transmitters, and bears a resemblance to certain slow-virus conditions. Like extrapyramidal syndrome it may therefore represent a final common path.

The longstanding distinction between "presenile" and "senile" forms of atrophic dementia is now no longer supportable, since the curve of incidence is continuous and shows no sign of bimodality[1] and the two forms are genetically associated.[1,2] The symptom-complex would best be referred to as Alzheimer's syndrome or alzheimerism, on the analogy of parkinsonism. It is characterized by progressive dementia focusing primarily on associative and recall processes, the presence of characteristic plaques and tangles, and cortical atrophy—now visible in life by tomographic scanning—due to massive loss of neurones.[3,4]

In fact, the natural histories of alzheimerism and of parkinsonism are remarkably similar. Each appears to have genetic determinants,[5] though not as marked as the genetic preferences of scrapie in sheep. If it were not for the recognition of the postencephalitic form, parkinsonism could well have been regarded as a "senile" or self-explanatory process with a "presenile" form reflecting genetic bad luck. Indeed, plaques and tubular tangles indistinguishable from those of Alzheimer's disease oc-

145

cur in postencephalitic parkinsonism, but in the nigral and cerulean neurones, not the hippocampus and cortex.[6] Parkinsonian dementia of Guam, in which rigidity and dementia occur usually without tremor, occupies a place intermediate between the other two classical syndromes, but closer to the atypical, tremorless parkinsonism of old age, which is eventually dementing in many cases. This disease, which causes about 7 per cent of deaths among native-born Chamorro Guamese, looks well-placed for an epidemiological attack like that mounted against kuru, but the small size of the population may obscure the fact that the cumulative incidence of alzheimerism in older Americans is almost certainly the same or greater.

These similarities in natural history do not indicate that alzheimerism and parkinsonism are "one disease," or that either has a unitary etiology, but they suggest a common nosology—one in which loss of strategically placed neurones is accompanied by defect in particular neurotransmitters: basal ganglia cells and dopamine in one case, cortical and hippocampal cells and acetylcholine in the other. Nor is it clear which comes first, the cell loss or the chemical defect, since the cortical cell loss may conceivably be trophic. The limited success in controlling parkinsonism certainly opens up the possibility of a similar attack on alzheimerism if the analogy holds true. Of the two, we know far less about alzheimerism, simply because it has been mistaken for an inherent manifestation of old age.

As in parkinsonism, some forms of alzheimerism may result directly from viral infection, either persistent, or acting by way of sensitization of immune mechanisms to brain cell protein.[7,8] In Huntington's chorea and Parkinson's disease the changes are localized in the striatum and the substantia nigra, respectively, whereas in Alzheimer's disease the mischief is hippocampal and cortical, and there is accumulating evidence that presynaptic acetylcholinergic fibers are chiefly involved.[9] The designation "senile" is philosophically unjustified except as a descriptive term, since although a few plaques may be observed in most brains of very old subjects, alzheimerism as a definite syndrome is not. Huntington's chorea, which is also a genetically determined abiotrophy with a long latent period, would have been regarded as senile if its latency had been substantially longer.

The genetic association of alzheimerism in relatives of patients with Down's syndrome and with hematologic malignancy[1] is interesting because subjects with Down's syndrome commonly develop Alzheimer-like changes at an early age and are at high risk from leukemias. Microtubular disorganization has been suggested as a common basis, on the ground that it too is increased by aging processes.[1] Leakage of tubule protein with the eventual appearance of autoimmunity is another possibility, while much work has been done on the association of alzheimerism with other chromosomal abnormalities.[10,11] In any analysis of the genetic basis of predisposition the high incidence in Down's syndrome is somewhat puzzling, since the risk to first-degree relatives of Down's syndrome patients, half of whom should inherit one defective gene, is low by comparison with expectation.

Choice between possible chain-of-event models is complicated by the virtual impossibility of prospective studies, but from a clinical point of view the most identifiable and potentially modifiable lesion appears to be a massive decline in choline acetyltransferase (CAT) and acetylcholinesterase (ACE) in the hippocampus, amygdala and cortex.[9,12] It is possible that this change directly reflects loss of either cells or synapses. On the other hand, judging from the results in palliating parkinsonism by the supply of deficient dopamine, attempts to supply acetylcholine or to reduce its degradation seem abundantly justified. Choline supplied in the diet had no striking effect on the dementing process[13] but since far higher and more sustained blood levels can be achieved with dietary lecithin,[14] this would appear to be the test material of first choice.[15] Missing from the present armamentarium is any serviceable ACE inhibitor not disqualified by its peripheral toxicity which could serve as part of a replacement-conservation or a replacement-neutralization therapy analogous to the combination of levodopa and carbidopa. If centrally-selective ACE inhibitors exist they might be sought among the compounds examined during the development of "irreversible" ACEI's for use as insecticides, or even war gases, but no therapeutic agent of this kind is now available.[16] The low levels of ACE present in Alzheimer brain are no bar to this approach—they may reflect a reduced number of synaptic sites, but they may equally be a response to low AC levels, a possibility which could be checked if AC levels would be raised substantially in Alzheimer patients.

A replacement approach would produce, on the most optimistic estimate, palliative results as good as those achieved with levodopa in parkinsonism, with arrest or partial regression of the dementing process.

The chief ground for therapeutic optimism is that in many cases of chronic brain syndrome (at least in the early stages) the dementing process is primarily an amnesia with which an otherwise fairly intact patient visibly wrestles. There is considerable resemblance between this process of inaccessibility to recall and the confusional effects of anticholinergic drugs[17]: it may therefore be a matter of neurotransmitter deficit rather than of irrevocable cell loss. The growing recognition of acute symptomatic brain syndrome in older persons precipitated by infection, medication and disturbances of electrolyte balance, in which a symptomatology as severe or severer is reversible, makes an energetic therapeutic approach to chronic brain syndromes much more credible. It will not be known how much they can be palliated until we conduct some therapeutic experiments.

Substantial prophylaxis, too, is not an unreasonable hope. It would obviously require an extensive program of neuroendocrine and immunologic studies, preferable longitudinal and concentrated among subjects at apparent genetic risk, since the fundamental changes probably long precede the appearance of dementing symptoms. One way of monitoring early chemical or immune changes which foreshadow eventual Alzheimer's disease might be to look for them in the only population where eventual incidence is known, i.e., young subjects with Down's syndrome. As long as experiment is limited to harmless materials such as lecithin, there would seem to be no ethical objection to seeing what an attempt to elevate brain ACh levels does to the eventual incidence of Alzheimer-type pathology in Down's syndrome—or for that matter to the mental state of Down's syndrome in general, where attention has focused more on tryptophan and serotonin than on ACh metabolism.

Alzheimerism may well turn out to cover a number of pathologies, some of which, like postencephalitic and manganese-induced parkinsonism, will prove to be epidemiologically identifiable. Among nonviral environmental factors most geriatric psychiatrists would wish to look at alcohol as a precipitant, but at the moment direct comparison of drinking with nondrinking communities (Mormon, Pentecostal) is likely to be frustrated by lack of proper postmortem criteria. The brief interest in aluminum toxicity based on the finding of high levels of Al in demented brain[18] appears to have subsided: Al levels are high in senile brain generally and correlate with age rather than dementia.[19] Environmental factors there certainly must be, however, judging from the existence of identical twins discordant for the disease.[20] Proper geriatric diagnosis and the demise of the shotgun diagnosis of "senility" to cover all confusional disorders of older people may make epidemiological research easier, but there is more than one dementing process in older people; at present there is no substitute for histological examination to differentiate alzheimerism with certainty.

Although the likelihood is that Alzheimer's disease is another complex and elusive process like multiple sclerosis involving immune, genetic, and possibly infective elements in close interplay, there is also the possibility of a far simpler biochemical lesion involving the inter-action of vasoactive peptides with the cholinergic system, the model proposed by Bowen.[12] This possibility can only become clearer with the present rapid advance in our knowledge of peptide neurohor-mones: for the present it might serve to focus attention on some of the features of alzheimerism other than the dementia—the cachexia which may accompany it, for example, and possible changes in hypothalamic rather than cortical function. The major attitudinal advance has al-ready taken place, however, in the recognition of late-life cerebral degeneration as a specific, common, and catastrophic disease, the pal-liation of which would alter the entire image of aging in the public mind.

REFERENCES

1. Heston, L.L. and Mastri, A.R.: The genetics of Alzheimer's disease. Arch. Gen. Psychiat. 34:976-981, 1977.

2. Sjogren, T., Sjogren, H. and Lundgren, A.G.H.: Morbus Alzheimer and morbus Pick: a genetic, clinical and neuroanatomic study. Acta psychiat. neurol. Scand., suppl. 82, 1963.

3. Bowen, D.M., Smith, C.B., White, P., Goodhardt, M.J., Spillane, J.A., Flack, R.H.A. and Davison, A.N.: Chemical pathology of the organic dementias, I. Brain 100: 397-426, 1977.

4. Bowen, D.M., Smith, C.B., White, P., Flack, R.H.A., Carrasco, L., Gedye, J.L. and Davison, A.N.: Chemical pathology of the organic dementias, II. Brain 100: 427-454,1977.

5. Martin, W.E., Loewenson, R.B., Resch, J.A. and Baker, A.B.: Parkinson's disease: clinical analysis of 100 patients. Neurology (Minn.) 23: 783-790,1973.

6. Wisniewski, H.M., Terry, R.D. and Hirano, A.: Neurofibrillary pathology. J. Neuropathol. Exp. Neurol. 29: 163-176, 1970.

7. Jankovic, B.D., Jakulic, S. and Horvat, J.: Cerebral atrophy, an immuno-logical disorder? Lancet ii:219-220, 1977.

8. Gajdusek, D.C.: Slow and latent viruses in the aged nervous system. In Maletta, G.J.: Survey report on the aging nervous system. DHEW NIH 74-296, 1974, pp. 149-162.

9. Davies, P. and Maloney, A.J.F.: Selective loss of central cholinergic neu-rons in Alzheimer's disease. Lancet ii:1403, 1976.

10. Jarvik, L.F.: Mental function related to chromosome findings in the aged. Amsterdam, Excerpta Medica, Series 274, 1974, pp. 851-855.

11. Jarvik, L.F., Altschuler, K.Z., Kato, T. and Blumner, B.: Organic brain syn-drome and chromosome loss in aged twins. Dis. Nerv. Syst. 32:159-170, 1971.

12. Bowen, D.M.: Biochemistry of dementias. Proc. Roy. Soc. Med. 70:351-352, 1977.

13. Boyd, W.D., Graham-White, J., Blackwood, G., Glen, I. and McQueen, J.: Clinical effects of choline in Alzheimer senile dementia. Lancet ii:711, 1977.

14. Wurtman, J.R., Hirsch, M.J., and Growdon, J.H.: Lecithin consumption raises serum-free-choline levels. Lancet ii:68,1977.

15. Perry, E.K., Perry, R.H. and Tomlinson, B.E.: Dietary lecithin supplements in dementia of Alzheimer type? Lancet ii:242-243, 1977.

16. Comfort, A.: Drug therapy in Alzheimer's disease. Lancet, 1978.

17. Drachman, D.A.: Human memory and the cholinergic system. Arch. Neurol. 30:113-121, 1974.

18. Crapper, D.R., Krishnan, S.S. and Dalton, A.J.: Brain aluminum distribution in Alzheimer's disease and experimental neurofibrillary degeneration. Science 180:511-513, 1973.

19. McDermott, J.R., Smith, A.I., Iqbal, K. and Wisniewski, H.M.: Aluminum and Alzheimer's disease. Lancet ii:710-711, 1977.

20. Hunter, R.A., Dayan, A.D. and Wilson, J.: Alzheimer's disease in one monozygotic twin. J. Neurol. Neurosurg. Psychiat. 35:707-10, 1972.

On Gerontophobia

Why do some doctors dislike the old? Not the hale and independent aged who look good for another twenty years; such old people give most of us a feeling of well-being that supports the image we like to entertain of our own eventual aging. The ones whom we fear and dislike are those who deface the image—the ailing, the crazy, and those who are about to die.

We may compensate for our feelings by jollying or patronizing the old folks. Our manner may be that which an anti-Semite, ashamed of his prejudice, adopts toward his Jewish friends. In both cases the falsity comes through.

In twenty years of attempting to interest medical and lay people in the welfare of the old, including the effort to build up geriatrics to palliate their troubles and fundamental gerontology to tackle the control of the aging process in the future, I had known that here was a subject in which there was a big unconscious load. I recognized it in myself, and it took no special insight to detect it in the literature.

The history of rejuvenation cures from Brown-Séquard onward—their involvement with potency magic, with the old human fantasy of living and being lovable forever—is a plain enough warning. It is difficult now to get a sensible reassessment, for instance, of the uses of testosterone in solid contexts like the control of osteoporosis or muscle loss. The subject has been so muddied by past attempts to use it as a resexualizing agent, and by the castration fears of generations of doctors and patients, that the judicious tend to consider the substance itself disreputable and its investigators as borderline quacks.

A more subtle disturbance is found in our attitude toward geriatric practice and research. The idea of doing anything about old age rings an alarm in the sober Anglo-American mind. People who work in geriatrics do so, whether they realize it or not, with the deep-seated wish to banish the knowledge that they themselves will age. The less critical or the overenthusiastic rush into print with great discoveries—chimpanzee testicles, procaine. The Great Tradition—our sort of medicine—rightly frowns on such enthusiasms; we leave them to irresponsible foreigners. At all costs we have to keep our unconscious involvement under firm control. The experimental biologist and the pure research man, like the artist in our society, is encouraged to develop fantasies;

he can speculate freely about the eventual control of aging, as he can about the eventual fathering of babies by dead geniuses or about the creation of new living forms. We, the clinicians, have to stay on the ground for the sake of our patients and our practices.

Accordingly, while we may endeavor to alleviate the ills of the aged, we are culturally required in undertaking the experiment to make it clear that we have little or no hope of succeeding. To admit the fantasy would be to accept the possibility of failure, leaving a raw surface in the mind. This we carefully guard against. Better still, we opt right out.

I recall being uneasy as a student when teacher after teacher explained that therapy was pointless or operation unnecessary because the patient was old, had had his time, could not expect miracles, and so on. Some moved the age of expendability far forward: at fifty-five or sixty the genital system became expendable ("he or she won't need it now"); at sixty-five further therapy was to be limited to encouragement. The image of later life was that of the well-behaved, asexual, uncomplaining subject, patiently awaiting the next world, to be kept as a pet if cheeringly vigorous, if not, to be jollied and avoided.

One sometimes sensed a wish that those among the elderly who failed to conform to the fantasy could be "put down," horse-fashion. Some senior teachers—themselves often close to sixty—adopted this line, and for all of them it was in striking contrast to their usual humane concern for people. Sometimes the two attitudes mixed: it was kinder to leave the old alone, which, where youthful officiousness was suggesting endless investigation or surgery, was quite true.

What I had not realized was the depth of aggression, however well controlled, that the prospect of irremediable illness stirs in medical men. It was brought home to me when I attended a seminar at which all the participants were senior practitioners directly and actively concerned with old people. The meeting was addressed by a woman who specialized in the care of the dying in a religious institution. She had devoted herself to helping the incurably sick to face and talk about the prospect of death and to accept it cheerfully. Her talk was illustrated with color slides of terminal patients, all smiling from the nose down.

The effect of this recital was a profound disturbance to the calm of everyone present. Having unintentionally broken down defenses right and left, she went on to ask directly: "Why do doctors avoid the dying? Why do they leave the deathbed to the nursing staff?" Before we could recover, she answered her own question with the anecdote of an old lady who said, "Doctor, you won't turn me out if I can't get better?"

The presentation which was given, I felt, without full insight on the part of the speaker, was psychiatrically catastrophic to the listeners. The seminar turned into a group therapy session. It had been a long time since I had seen deans of medical schools and senior physicians so upset. Some interpretation was clearly needed; one couldn't let them go home like that. Admitting hostility to one's patient is a hard enough lesson for the psychiatrist. It is one few physicians can readily live with.

And yet the experience, even without full interpretation, was highly beneficial to all. The clue to our disturbance had in fact been given—inadvertently—by the speaker. One of the exercises imposed upon her terminal patients was that they should frankly discuss their own impending deaths, so that visiting students could learn not to be embarrassed by mortality. One felt, however, that unless the students were to be given an opportunity to discuss their own feelings in the matter, there might well be repercussions.

When we enter medicine, we are adolescent or at least young. We come from a culture in which death is actively concealed, or if it is celebrated, the celebration amounts to a denial of Egyptian proportions. It is part of a physician's experience to be pitched straight into the physical, visual, and tactile recognition of death as a real and personal event while he is still immature and without (in most schools) any support in handling his own reactions. Most students are upset by it (whether the deathbed or the postmortem room upsets them the more will depend on their own anxieties). Some become depressed; a few drop out. Most acquire one or another kind of armor, which, in its developed form, is part of their professional equipment. At the outset the armor may be heartiness and realism; later it fuses with the discovery that there are people who can be helped, and that this is what activist medicine and surgery are all about. Death is tolerable to the doctor because he can sometimes postpone it. He deals with the idea of his own mortality, as most of us do, by repressing it as something a long way ahead. He responds to the idea of other peoples' deaths with activism. Medicine becomes a contest, with the physician or surgeon in the role of St. George.

This kind of carapace serves most of us well, unless we are disturbed or thin-skinned, and it has served medicine for many years. Its inadequacy appears only today, when the need to learn psychiatric attitudes the new way puts a low valuation on paternalism and omnipotence as medical postures, although our fathers adopted them without shame, and some of us still do. It is still chiefly the psychiatrist who hammers into students the idea that their self-estimate must include the knowledge that there are patients who cannot be magically made happy, problem-free, and euphoric, either by drugs or by interviews. Our patients give us every temptation to become gods or parents; it is only in psychiatry that we are seriously trained to resist this demand or to employ it insightfully.

For the ordinary clinician, it is the old or the dying person who shatters the protective stance. He is going to get worse, and we cannot stop him. Furthermore he is going to die, and so, one day, are we. Our divinity and paternity are fantasies, which he exposes. How dare he! We have learned to protect ourselves against an ultimate threat by asserting that we are different—we can help. The patient who obstinately gets worse and dies is doubly threatening. He castrates, or frustrates, us by denying our self-image as dragon slayers in round and tangible terms. At the same time he reminds us equally roundly that we too age and die. The aggression generated by such an attack on our identity is great, and the only available lightning conductor is the patient himself.

I feel quite sure this projected aggression is the answer to many questions about the embarrassment and bad faith that one so often senses in our approach to the man or woman who "cannot get well." It is a special and specially traumatic instance, with lesser parallels in our attitude to other "unsatisfactory" patients: the neurotic who cannot be made magically happy, the person with a chronic skin condition who cannot be healed like Naaman the Syrian, out of hand.

A satisfactory patient is an ego-boosting patient: we know in our consciences that all patients ought to be satisfactory—because they are human—and that they are not. Provided we can do something active, even if the patient dies, the confrontation is avoided. Unfortunately we cannot yet *do anything active* about old age. We can either pretend to, and deceive ourselves from worthy and humane motives, as do the discoverers of rejuvenation cures, or we can try by science to find techniques that work. If we are optimists with secure personalities, we can do this without self-deception or pessimism. If we are thinner-skinned, we hesitate to try; failure, or the discovery that age processes are basically not modifiable in the foreseeable future, would castrate us again, with further loss of inner security. Hence the rather depressing outcome of so much humanely intended research on age problems.

It is striking, though not surprising, how often the pattern of endeavor, success, and failure in research is psychoanalytically determined. It is still more striking and still less surprising, given the huge submerged element of magic and counter-transference in the iceberg of clinical medicine, how slightly aware we are of what our patients do to us by ailing, recovering, or dying.

Aging, because it is progressive, threatens our adjustment. In the person of the old or dying patient there is a menacing Freudian equation with our own elders and fathers. If we are fathers, then he is the naughty child who impertinently steals our virility and identity. If we are medical gods, he is our devoted Adam. This is dangerous material, which we must either face or export. We usually do the second, by projecting it against the patient. That, I submit, is why our seminar made us all feel uneasy.

The prescription for our unease before the old, before aging, and before death (in a culture that is talking quite seriously of deep-freezing the dying against the time of a magical resurrection) is the same as for all medical acting-out, the acquisition of insight—early in training if possible, but later if necessary. In fact it should be early, the earlier the better. The establishment of a program of group sessions to continue from the start of medical education, directed to teaching the biology of human relations, and incidentally and simultaneously, to giving the student supportive insight into his own experience of becoming a physician, could cut the dropout and psychiatric breakdown rate among students. And of course it could also give us much better doctors.

The modern student, imbibing radiation biology, therapeutics, biochemistry, physics, and technologies innumerable, can easily take refuge from less manageable insights in a detailed knowledge of plasma electrolytes, thereby avoiding the painful acquisition of a more important technology, that of the emotions and of being a person. Good clinicians of the old school knew this intuitively and handled it by insight; it is the skill that distinguishes the physician from all other technologists. Research men need it no less: their unconscious motives are reflected in their choice of research, and their limitations spring from emotionally loaded topics like aging. If our culture requires more insight into the unconscious origins of all of its apparently hard-core activities, from space travel to freezing corpses—both of them shamanic ventures of great human antiquity—the serious scientific control of human aging processes, which is well within the bounds of realistic venture, demands a similar degree of emotional insight, if for no more than the hope of mere practical success.

Without insight we get monkey glands on one hand and self-defeating timidity on the other. The experience of looking hard at our attitudes can be very unpleasant, as the seminar showed us, but unless we undertake it we shall neither treat our old patients with integrity, nor realize the perfectly worthy human fantasy of postponing death and decay.

V

On Human Biology

Is Sociobiology Real?

Science progresses both by discoveries and by fads. The fads fade, but may, if handled properly, leave some solid insights behind them. "Sociobiology" is not a new but a recurrent fad. In its original form it derives its ancestry from primitive man, which anthropomorphized animals (usually, however, in a much more sophisticated way than the zoo visitor who thinks of apes or pandas as little people, but at the same time is quite content to see them confined under unbiological conditions). Philosophy from the Greeks onward set man apart on the ground of rationality—a perfectly correct division, we now know, because it turns upon the nongenetic, nonrandom character of social as against biologic evolution. Eastern philosophy was less certain, on transmigrationist grounds, and more interested in human ways of seeing than in a rigidly objectivized universe, physical or biological—an insight, too, that is coming into its own.

It was the 19th century which reversed the intuition of the primitive by developing a theromorphic view of man rather than an anthropomorphic view of animals. It did so in a manner in keeping with its manipulative view of the universe—brash, selfjustificatory, and often ignorant of actual animal behaviors. We have every reason, living in the wash from that period of entrepreneurial bumptiousness and commercial imperialism, to look on revivals of "sociobiology" with intense suspicion. Neo-Darwinisms have a way of being adopted, like the Marseillaise or the Flag, by extremists of the right or the left bent on propaganda. Moreover, since nothing allays anxiety about ourselves like the assurance that our unbiddable impulses or needs are in some way natural and built-in, genetic determinism is raided to yield us consolation. The subject, in fact, is a mess.

The specific revival of the term "sociobiology" at the present time we owe to Wilson.[1,2] His work, though not immune to the pitfalls of extrapolation from instinctual to culturally-transmitting animals, is intellectually distinguished: some of the abuse it has incurred has been due less to what he has said than to anxiety about what less intelligent or critical diadochi might make of it. This is not a legitimate ground for attack, but in view of the history of the subject, comprehensible, as we shall see. Probably his most important single point for psychiatric readers is a restatement in plain of the biologic importance of the expansion of reproduction in Man into sexuality—something seen only in primates, where the "hypertrophy" of what were phylogenetically mating behaviors into bonding, under the influence of constant female receptivity, explains a number of paradoxes; for example, the ability of males to erotize males, which is reproductively disadaptive but socially adaptive. This is not a new point, in view of the work of writers like Zuckerman and Sahlins, which is now twenty years old; but the concept of hypertrophy is particularly felicitous. For other human biopsychological effects we really need a mirror term to cover examples such as pheromone excitation, where the apparatus and pathways appear to be there, but the practical and behavioral importance is larval because more complex behaviors have in most contexts taken over, the result being not atrophy (which would be the complement of Wilson's hypertrophy) but behavioral override. What hypertrophy is apparently species-determined in Man and built into phylogeny. What is overridden differs strikingly from culture to culture. Moreover, since the overridden pathways persist they remain identifiable. Incest, against which Wilson postulates a phylogenetic "gut feeling," is a difficult case. It would be unsurprising if there were indeed a built-in behavioral avoidance, but, as Freud pointed out, social taboos would in that event be unnecessary. It is not clear whether genetic promiscuity is the free-running condition, as in most primates, and exogamy the result of the "override," or whether our unavailable ancestors had genetic scruples, but cultural and individual intellection tends to override these on occasion. One suspects that in the fuss over a disturbing behavior we are missing the point—that what is both inbuilt and idiosyncratic in Man is the ability of the male to identify, and respond ambivalently to, immature males on the sight of genitalia, not secondary sex characters, so that the "Edipal reaction" is a built-in temporary organ like the tadpole's tail, directed to prevent over-reaction within the family, and not, as Freud imagined, a racial reminiscence of a horde situation in which father and son fought for mates.

The fact that Freud has acquired intense interest for primatologists at precisely the time when his therapeutic importance seems to be waning suggests a large area of genuine sociobiology which could be profitably opened if psychoanalysts and ethologists more often read one another's papers. This view of the uses of biological retrospect in human psychogenesis gives us some notion of the difficulty of gauging the interplay between hypertrophy, overriding, and idiosyncratic learning. Other areas of sexual behavior—notably "releasers" and the overdetermination of sexual fetishes—present similar questions. Does imprinting occur in Man? If so, he is quite unusual among altricial animals. If imprinting occurs, is it ever hormonally slanted by the prenatal environment, e.g., in the case of gender roles? The overwhelming probability, if one were betting, is that all questions on biological heritage versus override require *both/and,* not *either/or* answers, which is why ideological zealots make bad sociobiologists. *Both/and* is not in their mode of thinking.

The first distinction to be made, however, is between legitimate sociobiology, which is what Wilson espouses, and what is better called barroom biology—the naive application to man of theromorphic analogies based (usually) on a minimal or inaccurate knowledge of biology wedded to a self-justificatory or ideological purpose. The progress of eugenics into *Rassenheilkunde,* the notion of "biologically fixed" sex roles which it is "abnormal" to ignore, or the argument that, "Since I am consumed with aggression and certain animals are in certain circumstances aggressive, aggression is 'natural' to man," are among the most familiar examples. Closely related is the attempt to biologize racism. This, however, is of a slightly different order, because it represents the GIGO principle ("garbage in, garbage out") as it affects science. If a social posture or any other type of vulgar prejudice is taken as an axiom, and tests or experiments are based on its unrecognized or self-evident assumptions, garbage will result. While barroom biology begins in ignorance—of the real behaviors of primates, for example, which are only now being observed, and are far from anthropomorphic, or in ignorance of the difference between instinct and the capacity to acquire social programming—GIGO formulations depend on unrecognized assumptions. There is a GIGO element in a great deal of legitimate science, which makes its use in the legitimation of irrational behaviors particularly dangerous. Even our natural assumption of an "objective" universe distinct from the human mode of perceiving and processing phenomena is an element of preconception which physics and neuropsychology have only transcended when forced to do so by their own logic. Since all human ratiocination begins in a brain which has been formed by learning, all hypotheses embody prejudices, and much of the knack of science lies in devising means of circumventing them by "thinking against" the brain.[3]

Sometimes genuine scientific insights depend on a climate of social attitude to make them possible; not only do capitalist eras tend to produce those (otherwise validable) hypotheses which might occur to a capitalist mind, and marxist societies those which might be expected to occur to a marxist, but acceptance, even after initial controversy and choice of the agenda for speculation are grossly determined by society. Ideas of evolution, of a structured pattern in irrational behaviors, and of an analogy between mechanics and cosmology have often appeared, as it were, in orbit, but for them to be plucked down and elaborated by a Darwin, a Freud or a Newton required a social climate which might criticize but still facilitated the exercise. Originals like Blake, who attempt to deny current phenomenology, get driven out of science into art, or become "sleepers" for later rediscovery. The real distinction of GIGO sociobiology, as against serious biopsychological comment, and also of GIGO psychiatry, sexology, or genetics is that the bad faith is partially evident to its creators, who not infrequently (like Cyril Burt, the originator of racial intelligence testing) are found retrospectively to have resorted to fraud in producing results. Writers of the standing of Wilson do not deserve to be tarred with this brush, but it explains the anxiety with which the title "sociobiology" has been invested among many.

Fake sociobiology in America has been largely concerned with validating racism. Fake sociobiology in Britain was chiefly directed to prove the unfitness for responsibility of the "working class." Fake sociobiology in the Soviet Union attempted the equivalent of a reverse takeover to demonstrate Lamarckian inheritance in the biological realm. In so doing it painted itself into a corner, for it is far easier to fake social than biological data, and the implications of falsification had immediate repercussions in agriculture. Not all pseudobiological comment in human affairs is so patently manipulative, however. Much of it is made in good faith out of the strength of the temptation to generalize. The gross examples—such as Dr. Stockard's famous venture in which he crossed a beagle with a St. Bernard and took the progeny on a lecture tour to illustrate the evils of human miscegenation—are not the most misleading.

Since sociobiology as a concern is bound to return every few years, a proper approach to renewed interest and renewed production of popular books is the examination of what a biological approach to social phenomena could achieve if it were done conscientiously and competently. The mere attempt to do this is a valuable exercise in the science of science. The fact that it has been done before by writers such as Haldane, Waddington and Medawar, does not lessen the need to repeat the lesson: the likely gains are just as much in our understanding of biology through society as the other way around.

It is evident that Man, being an animal, has a biology. Men tend to be physically stronger than women, they are unable to give birth to or suckle infants, and their role in sexuality depends on erection and intromission. Accordingly there are "biological" invariants through which the experiences, and hence some of the attributes, of men and women must differ. This, however, does not affect the fact that "sex roles," and even more remarkably gender roles, in humans are demonstrably learned, and that the override from learning can transcend, or at least seriously confuse, genetic, hormonal and anatomical determination. In Man biology exists, but its most salient feature is that in human biology *the override from learning takes precedence.* Thus elaborate systems demonstrable in lower primates which determine aspects of their behavior are demonstrable in humans, but have lost much of their primacy, or are diverted into an unfamiliar function. Thus pheromones play a large part in the mating and cyclicity of monkeys. Humans retain the complete equipment, including olfactosexual reactions and probably pheromonal influences on cyclicity, but the primacy of the system has been replaced by other signals of a social kind (males do not become impotent like monkeys when female secretions are altered by "the pill"), and the pheromone responses may possibly have become diverted into special functions connected with infantile sexuality.[4] Footballers now congratulate a winner in a manner reminiscent of rejoicing among chimpanzees, but they only began to do so recently, as inhibitions on male-male demonstrative behaviors were relaxed, and then only in some cultures. Britain has witnessed the spread of a similar primate congratulatory ritual into cricket. The "biology" may have been there, but it has only now been let out.

One important rule of "sociobiology" would therefore appear to be that where humans can be shown to share in some system which in lower primates determines behavior, that system is likely at most to function as one of a number of overdeterminants where human behaviors are involved, and the size of its contribution will be reduced in proportion to the complexity of those behaviors. This, of course, applies to systems seen in the total setting, not to anatomical systems or neuroendocrine "bits." The mechanisms involved in expressing, say, rage may well be the same in man and in other mammals, and the neuroendocrine events similar (rather as both man and other mammals which possess teeth use them in biting) but the triggering, expression, and social contexts of this piece of final common path behavior are formed in man predominantly by the override from learning.

Indeed, all of the major biological idiosyncrasies of man seem to group themselves around learning ability and increased brain size. They range from the long period of infantile dependence and the complications arising from "infantile sexuality" in its Freudian sense, where competitive reactions normally triggered by the secondary sex characters have been transferred to the genitalia and used to structure quite a different process, namely individuation,[5] to the unusually long human lifespan with its postreproductive period. By Pangloss' Theorem we can see that all these things "must be so." A preprogrammed and prewired human brain would have been too big to go through a pelvis compatible with the erect posture, and brains in general—even in kittens—are not as a rule prewired, but rather formed by experiential inputs which delete connections and reinforce others. The notion of human "instincts," if such were ever demonstrable, subsisting in neural structure is improbable. "Instinctual" constants such as motherlove, altruism or its reverse, and sexual appetency are far more likely, if genuine, to be chemical, or based on an interplay between a chemical invariant common to mammals and neural programming by experience. It is significant that the most striking analogy to the lock-and-key instinctual rigidity of animals is found in Man among behaviors which are slightly atypical, such as the fixity of sexual fetishes. Neurologists have had much play with the "grandmother cell" or "grandmother circuit" which in pre-holographic models was postulated to localize our recognition of our grandmother. If grandmother-recognition were really built-in, one would now look for a grand-mother-molecule which triggers behavior appropriate to such a recognition, because that at least would be compatible with the space-constraints imposed by the fetal skull.

It is unfortunate, too, that even proficient and innovative sociobiology chronically tends, whenever it is rediscovered, to combine postures based on biology as it was some years previously with unripe enthusiasm for very recent investigations (primate ethology is the latest of these) without any grasp of the breadth of intermediate development in the subject. It is incredibly difficult for one theorist to know all the necessary disciplines. Much of what is written about evolutionary genetics in this field today is without benefit of recent development in the subject—usually because it is written by non-biologists, or biologists whose compartmentalized interests exclude an overview. This makes it—or rather, the moderation of its excesses—a highly suitable field for "higher studies," in that no single area—genetics, evolution, behavioristic psychology—can talk unmischievous sense without benefit of the others (as well as of anthropology, psychoanalytic psychology, art history, computer theory, and—though it is not a discipline—a modicum of common sense, singularly lacking from the most popular writings on the subject). It is much simpler to develop a "shtik"—it all depends on inheritance, or on territoriality, or on some hasty observations on baboons. Of such stuff bestsellers are most readily moulded.

So much for spurious sociobiology—what of the genuine? There probably is more serious and, if one may use the word, decent, work in the area of human social biology today than there has been for a long time. Both Wilson and some of his successors are acutely aware of the kind of unedifying generalization to which I have referred. Many are heroic enough to tackle difficult areas. A recent book by Symons[8] is a model of how sociobiological theories can be presented. The material—innate versus cultural differences between men and women—is obviously real: some of the differences under study, being structural, can hardly be a matter of dispute. But once we leave this tangible area, the trouble begins. Is the tag about the polygamous male and the monogamous female a folk-observation about human frailty, or a statement about human biology? Is jealousy a cultural convention or analogous to the behaviors of bulls and roosters? Do female animals other than human females exhibit orgasm, and if not, why have we evolved it? Now the sociobiologist's standard method of dealing with these issues is comparative (he looks at animals, and reads the reports of ethnographers) and then, when he has established the prevalence of a behavior in humans, Panglossian—he looks for the possible adaptive history of the status quo. Symons does all this with a straight face, and then indicates that he recognizes the methodological bind by giving a plausible evolutionary-adaptive history for a phenomenon (retention of estrus) which does not occur in humans. If it did, sociobiologists would use exactly this argument to explain it. This is very like dealing with your analyst by offering an entirely different but equally Freudian interpretation of a dream which he has just interpreted. Symons, too, has a sense of humor, and recognizes that "primitives" in their dealings with impertinent strangers have sometimes had one, too. The anthropological discourses on the sexual behaviors of alien people, snippets from which embellish all sociobiological treatises worth the name, are sometimes observational, usually nonparticipatory, and not infrequently mere gossip. Even in our own society it is hard to establish what attitudes really are. Even Symons assumes it to be true that males, if they have any inherent attitude, tend to be jealous. Is this in the direct line of bulls, roosters and some primates, or not? One could see adaptive reasons for it, though as Symons points out, the angry cuckold is not unconsciously defending the transmission of his genes. In fact, given some of the unconventional situations which our society tolerates, a different observer might well emphasize that so far from making enemies, sharing a woman creates brothers-by-adoption, and does so in species where two males then ally themselves to out-threaten single rivals. In drafting any sociobiological hypothesis, it would be wise first to consult some of the most skilled observers. (I would pick Tolstoy and Shakespeare.) Karenin's ambivalent encounter with Anna's lover? Othello screwing himself up to display the jealousy which the culture expects? Or the husbands one meets in our society, who greet the occasional wifely infidelity with relief because it reduces conjugal ammunition against their own philandering? Psychoanalysts have long interpreted wife exchange and the affinity which results from it as homosexual by surrogation—in other words, as reinforcing male-male bonding. One is tempted to turn even Symons' cautious argument round and see women as the biologically adapted creators and men as the victims of "jealousy"—but that too would founder in the wealth of human overdetermination. And indeed, having run the whole course, and pointed out that man and woman must and do differ, Symons himself sets the record straight in a passage which should be a condition of probation for all those convicted of half-baked biosocial formulation:

There are, I believe, several general implications in the line of reasoning pursued here. First, data, not theory and not analogies with nonhuman animals, reveal what human beings are like. Second, evolutionary analyses must consider the question of the environments for which organisms have been designed, however speculative such consideration may be. Structures, behaviors, and psyches that develop in unnatural environments may not have ultimate causes at all. Third, the tendencies to equate "natural" and "good" and to find dignity in biological adaptation can only impede understanding of ultimate causation and distort perceptions of nonhuman animals, preliterate peoples, and history. Finally, the *potentials* of a biological mechanism are not necessarily constrained by, and cannot necessarily be predicted from, the *purposes* for which the mechanism was designed by natural selection. Perhaps it is not excessively naïve to hope that a creature capable of perceiving the plowshare in the sword is also capable of freeing itself from the nightmare of the past.[8]

On that statement it would be difficult for anyone to improve.

Is there, then, any genuine discipline we can or should call "sociobiology"?

I have referred already to Wilson.[1,2] He has made a case for his title, but in fact the majority of serious comparative study needs no special title, for it falls either under the rubric of biology or that of human biology. It might have been wiser to adopt no special disciplinary banner. The instructive—and novel—area which perhaps really merits a distinctive title is not the comparison of man with animals, but the comparison of human activities with biological systems, and this had not yet been addressed. Consider the "sociobiology" of costume. Animal forms, plumage, pigmentation, and morphology generally, are the product of evolution. Human costume is the product of social choice, subject to only the evident ecological constraints of climate and available technology. Yet if we apply to costume the same analysis of function which we would use if it were genetically determined, we find examples of mimicry, cryptism, dominance signalling, sexual releasers, superstimuli, convergence, special adaptation, and indeed most of the phenomena displayed by animal interspecific and intersexual variation. This variation, moreover, is analogous, not homologous, because it is the product of an "evolution" which is social, Lamarckian and noetic, with a repertoire of "innate" factors serving as pegs on which it is hung, but in which the major development is socially transmitted—yet the convergence on animal variation is more than fanciful.

Where less visible and less simple human activities are examined, moreover, very similar convergence between social and biological "evolutions" can be made out. Convergence depends not on homology but on the constraints of function on variability. The comparison is accordingly valid. From this it follows that where in an evolved spectrum of activities particular niches have been filled, we can reasonably look for analogous products of social evolution.

The instructive part of this is not, however, the application of biological analogy to social evolution, but a more rigid critique of natural selection in its original, deterministic, context. Human social evolution, though it is not teleonomic, in the sense that its pretentions and aims are at variance with its overt results even at a primitive level, is undoubtedly noetic—it involves an element of ratiocination and purpose. Natural evolution, in the view of the vast majority of modern biologists, does not. Yet man has intense difficulty in holding consistently to any non-teleological picture of natural evolution because his entire experience in the far faster and more domestic timescale of social-Lamarckian evolution is of the teleological kind typical of man himself. Since we design hypotheses in language, which is the currency of the social mode, nonteleological evolutionary formulations are enormously cumbersome. It is far simpler as a rule to assume teleology and then correct the model. As a result a biologist may deliberately ask, "Why does this orchid need to simulate the female of a wasp with such precision? Could it not ensure fertilization in a less specific way?" We know, and he knows, that he does not mean exactly that, but it is simpler to reduce non-noetic interaction to the noetic level, simply as a shorthand. Most scientific attention has since Darwin been focussed on the analysis of the non-teleological natural process, simply because it had to be clearly discriminated from the anthropomorphic model. An argument for the existence of God would now have to be not an argument from design but an argument from the absence of design which nonetheless has generated the biological order. In the heat of the conflict with bigots a great many discontinuities in evolutionary theory at the biological level have been glossed over (not least the "acrostic paradox"—how one genetic "word" can transform in evolution to another without passing through prohibited nonsense combinations; and some of the incredibly precise coevolutive systems between host and parasite, flower and pollinator, where a readback in straightforward stochastic-selectionist terms is extremely difficult).

Full comprehension of an analogous system of variation and selection which is teleological, nonhereditary, and therefore several orders of magnitude faster in passing from one stable state to another, is instructive in our understanding of selectionist evolution simply because it is analogous, not homologous; and because language, human thought processes, and hypothesis-making are themselves heavily moulded by experience, not of natural evolution, which is a mental construct which took centuries to clarify, but of the familiar, teleological, social version. The building of biogenesis has four floors—atomic, molecular, biological-stochastic, and now, in man noetic. We had to work out the rules applying to the third floor with equipment tested on the fourth, and it has not been easy. We have invariably had to start, in Haldane's words, from Pangloss' Theorem, that everything has to be as it is to have gotten where we find it. There is accordingly a great deal which could be added to modern nonteleological bioevolutionary theory by a parallel study of the social, teleological milieu in which human development and social variation occur.

All post-Waddingtonian selectionist theory draws on this process of comparison as a way of revealing difference, but in the obligate concentration of biology on biological evolution the usefulness of the comparison has not yet been fully worked out.

Whether there is at the last word any underlying unity between noetic and non-noetic evolution is quite another thing: if there is it is likely to be at a further level of abstraction, not in any revival of neo-vitalism in a more sophisticated form, based on the idea that all problem-solving systems possess "mind-like" properties. What does appear to have happened is that biological evolution has by its own proper motion developed by stochastic variation and by selection biological systems able to short circuit the stochastic elements in itself, through a process of forward-looking stimulation using a developed nervous system. The fourth floor has been constructed by the third. With its construction, elements from the earlier mode—so popular with genetic apocalyptists—have become very largely irrelevant to man because of their infinitely longer timescale. We shall not "evolve" into leglessness through using motorcars, even if these render congenitally legless people able to survive, or any other such nonsense, but we may change ourselves by intervention, purposive or accidental, and *it is this mode which now constitutes the evolutionary biology of man.*

"What is important (for natural selection) is not survival, but the transmission of qualities to offspring...when we speak of those which survive, or better transmit, as being the fittest, we are really adding nothing to the statement that they transmit."[6] That the development of culturally transmitted variation is evolution, and not a mere copy or imitation of it in another universe of discourse, was clearly stated by Waddington over fifteen years ago. Since it is this dimension which is both social and characteristically human, it is odd that the emphasis of professing "sociobiology" is still on matters of vestigial genetic predisposition rather than on the aspect of human biology which is genuinely novel in phylogeny. The real interest of primate ethology is not that man and apes share some behaviors, but that the point of transition from genetic to cultural transmission of behaviors, and the remoulding of older automatisms by it, is as critical a systems break as biogenesis, and far more accessible to direct study. Indeed, the reason that "altruism" occupies so large a part in discussions of evolutionary effects on behavior is not that it is accessible to biometry, but that it is the basis on which sociality develops in social species. A social animal is one which displays the capacity to acquire behavioral programming by reading cues from conspecifics, or from surrogate conspecifics such as man when the animal is domesticated. With this capacity a dog rapidly acquires sensitivity to human language, a stimulus to which it would never be exposed in the wild: a cat, not being "social," does so only on a basis of conditioning. This is the phylogeny of cultural transmission, but its further development clearly depended on the develop-

168

ment of transmitting mechanisms: the social capacity of dogs resembles a CB radio in being sensitive to incoming signals over a far greater range than it is capable of transmitting. The time-sequence of enlarged brain, language, manipulative dexterity, and environmental pressures (change of habitat, climatic and migratory influences) has been debated from a fossil record which continues to grow. On most matters of anthropogenesis the jury is still out. But these areas of study, and this emphasis, are clearly very critical to a phylogenetic "sociobiology," and it will be rewarding to develop one.

Cultural evolution, in sum, is a continuous part of evolution, not a shadow, simulacrum or analogous model. It belongs in this sense to biology, and "sociobiology" is perhaps as good a term for this area of discourse as any other. It is, however, the antithesis of theromorphic social Darwinism, genetic determinism, and the general background of 19th and early 20th century biologism which has made the idea of "sociobiology" as suspect as that of "eugenics." Few charlatanisms have done as much harm as this one. One wonders what Hofstadter, who chronicled some of its influence, would have made of Shockley, Jensen and some more recent hierophants of genetic determinism.[7] Indeed, in order to get rid of the guilt by association we may be forced to get rid of the name. Yet there is or could be a sociobiology which is neither naive nor reactionary. The areas of study which I have outlined form a part of its agenda and have an importance for the understanding of human evolution, and evolution in general, by whatever name we elect to describe the study, which will long outlive the nominal creation of new disciplinary titles and the exploitation of pseudo-scientific fashion.

1. Wilson, E.D.: Sociobiology: The New Synthesis. Cambridge, Belknap Press (Harvard University Press), 1975.

2. Wilson, E.D.: On Human Nature. Cambridge, Belknap Press (Harvard University Press), 1978.

3. Bachelard, G.: Le nouvel esprit scientifique. Paris, 1949.

4. Comfort, A.: The likelihood of human pheromones. Nature 230:432-433, 1971.

5. Comfort, A.: Darwin and Freud. Lancet ii:107-111,1960.

6. Waddington, C.H.: The human evolutionary system. In Darwinism and the Study of Society (edited by Bantom M.) London, Tavistock, 1961.

7. Hofstadter, I.R.: Social Darwinism in American Thought. (Revised edition.) Boston, Beacon Press, 1955.

8. Symons, D. The evolution of human sexuality. Oxford University Press, 1979.

The Likelihood of Human Pheromones

A pheromone is a substance secreted by one individual which affects the behavior of another of the same species—an olfactory hormone.

Pheromones control ant behavior and much insect mating. An artificial pheromone (gyplure) can be synthesized to attract gypsy moth males into an insecticidal trap. Pheromones are also widespread in mammals. Some mammalian odors, like the n-butyl-mercaptan of the skunk, or the labelling of territory with urine, are straightforward signals. These influence behavior in the same way as a display of threat, dominance or attraction. The action of a true pheromone is more direct; it is a signal, but its action is more like that of a hormone—the distinction is not total, but it is perceptible, in that many pheromonal odors, at least in mammals, have a chemical shape rather like that of a steroid molecule, and might have been derived from one.

We are all familiar with mammalian examples of the signal type—the attraction of a bitch in season, or the rejection by a ewe of a lamb which "smells wrong" and is not her own. Pheromones may be "releasers" (straightforward signals of this kind) or "primers", which act by bringing about a receptive or appropriate state for future behavior—by synchronizing estrus cycles, for example. It is the second kind which are physiologically the more interesting in mammals.

The likelihood that there are functional human pheromones has been asserted (Wilson, 1963; Wiener, 1966, 1967a, 1967b) and denied (Gleeson and Reynierse, 1969), both without direct experimental evidence: the finding of clear pheromonal effects in monkeys (Michael and Saayman, 1967; Michael and Keverne, 1970) and the apparent observation of menstrual synchronization between close friends (McClintock, 1971) re-open the possibility more definitely, and make direct experiment obligatory.

The practical importance of such research lies in the possibility of primer control over human endocrine cycles and reproduction generally; if this exists, it might open a new chapter in reproductive pharmacology at a time when it is badly needed. Compared with drugs, pheromones are strikingly economical in quantity, many operating at a level of molecules rather than milligrams. Even the study of simple "releaser" effects could clarify a field of human, and especially developmental, biology which has been so far suspected rather than elucidated. Odor fingerprinting techniques and gas chromatography (Dravnieks and Krotoszynski, 1970) now make the detection and preparation of human pheromonal agents feasible if they exist.

Developmental Effects

Sexual releaser effects of odor in man have been recognized throughout human experience, even in cultures which found the idea embarrassing, and the richness of human olfactosexual behavior was fully documented by Havelock Ellis (1905). All releaser effects in man tend to be more variable than in lower animals because of the large variety of human signal systems and the size of the override from learned or conditioned behavior, which is such that not even the human sex object is irrevocably fixed. The large observed individual variation in conscious olfactory awareness is almost certainly in part genetic, but psychoanalytic writers have both suggested and documented the possibility of a special role for odor in infant psychosexual development (Brill, 1932; Daly and White, 1930; Bieber, 1959; Fitzherbert, 1959; Kalogerakis, 1963). According to this view, attraction to the odor of the opposite-sex parent and avoidance as a threat of the odor of the same-sex parent act as biological triggers for the Oedipal responses, an idea of much biological interest. This would represent a case intermediate between releaser and primer conditions, and possibly a programmed "temporary organ."

We have the observation of several workers, notably Kalogerakis (1963) and Bieber (1959) that odor plays an important part in infantile psychosexual development. The stage in development when dominance-competition between son and father appears, the "oedipal phase," is accompanied by a marked awareness of the sexual odor of adults, with a distaste for that of the same-sex parent. A biological psychoanalyst could not fail to note that three regions in man are provided with odor glands and large, odor-diffusing hair tufts—the breast-axilla complex, and the anal and genital regions, all imprinting points in human development. The odor of the areolar glands, which adults cannot perceive, could be our first impression in life. The sequence of associations is biologically interesting.

Groddeck (1925) argued that man is as macrosmatic as the dog, but represses the capacity in adult life for psychosexual reasons. Without accepting this view, it is still credible that some part of human olfactosexual response may be confined to infancy and childhood, and subsequently "turned off," or altered in direction, either by a process of repression or, as in other mammals, by the advent of adult sex hormone status, most adult pheromone response being either androgen or estrogendependent. The complexity of human psychosexual development is likely to produce unique effects on adult response not seen in other mammals. "Even the most learned man," said Groddeck, "has to let his nose decide for him in matters of love." For some people this is consciously true. Unfortunately for simple analysis, we tend to "imprint" releasers from past experience—musk, human or animal, is a "releaser," but so, for some people, is the odor of gasoline rubber, through a conditioned association with contraceptives. Babies can be readily conditioned to like the smell of cod liver oil (Welch and Hayes, 1957).

Adult Effects

Adult odor releaser effects in man as embodied in sexual behavior are attractant, ancillary to more familiar signal systems, and often overridden by individual experience, though still serving to synchronize intercourse with ovulation: beside male—female attraction, or bonding during pregnancy, they may possibly on the mammalian model, include adult male—male dominance or hostility. Wider odor communication of states of mind, as postulated by Wiener (1966), is ill-confirmed in other mammals and difficult to separate from other human subliminal cues. The value of seeking for the more tangible and important primer effects, which have not been suspected so far, depends on the following principal arguments:

1. Pheromonal primer effects are near-universal in social animals, including primates.

2. Releaser pheromone effects exist in man, at least in larval form, and some involve pheromones of other mammals (musk, civetone). These in nature are rarely simple releasers, but combine priming and other effects—thus one male odor may serve to mark territory, assert dominance, repel rivals, attract females and synchronize their cycles. Unless man is a wholly special case, or his use of this potential response system has been taken over by anticipation, as part of infantile rather than adult psychosexual mechanics, then similar effects are to be looked for in man also.

3. In mammals as against insects, functional and species specificities do not seem to depend on a multiplicity of special substances. Cross-specific reactions are common (humans react to musk; bulls, goats and

monkeys to the odor of women): interspecific bars between near species (dog—fox) are probably effected by addition or by concentration, the basic effector molecules being widespread. The physiological effect of similar molecules is likely to be similar between man and other mammals in which priming is known to occur.

4. Humans have a complete set of organs which are traditionally described as non-functional, but which, if seen in any other mammal, would be recognized as part of a pheromone system. These include apocrine glands associated with conspicuous hair tufts, some of which do not produce sweat and most presumably produce some other functioning secretion (Kligman and Shehadeh, 1964); a developed prepuce and labia, and the production of smegma (the sebaceous secretion that collects beneath the prepuce or around the clitoris). This system in adults seems over-elaborate for the relatively small releaser role of odor in most cultures. The amputatory assault on these recognizable pheromone-mediating structures in many human societies implies an intuitive awareness that their sexual function goes beyond the decorative. A conspicuous and apparently unused antenna array presupposes an unsuspected communications system.

Patterns of Response

The nature and function of such possible communications can be inferred from mammalian models to indicate the types of priming which might be expected in humans. For instance, Le Magnen (1952) showed that women's ability to smell musks varies with the estrus cycle. It is known that women have greater olfactory sensitivity to most mammal odor, that this is estrogen-dependent and in the case of exaltolide, cyclical (Kloek, 1961; Vierling and Rock, 1967). Thus women detect, and react to, boar taint in pork far more readily than men (Griffiths and Patterson, 1970), the substance detected being apparently 5α-androst-16-en-3-one (Patterson, 1968). A similar material occurs in human male urine, and in female urine during the luteal phase (Brookbank and Hazelwood, 1950).

The detection of this effect seems to depend on the choice of olfactometric method. According to Amoore (Amoore and Venstrom, 1966; Amoore, personal communication) there is no true change of threshold, but women under the influence of estrogen are more inclined to react psychologically to musky odors and to describe them as "strong."

True anosmia, both for a musk (pentadecalactone) and for iso-valeric acid, has been reported in man (Whissell-Buechy and Amoore, 1973). Musk anosmia was found in 7.2% of Caucasians but not in Black subjects; iso-valeric acid anosmia was found in 9.1% Blacks and 1.4% Caucasians. The anosmias are heritable, but the samples were not broken down by age, sex, or ingestion of hormones such as oral contraceptives. Anosmia for a potential pheromone is of biologic interest, but there is no evidence that iso-valeric acid anosmia, or the suppression of acid vaginal components by the Pill, overtly affect human sexual behaviors.

Since human male sexual behavior is non-cyclical and not dependent on female receptivity, the female>male influence may well be releaser only, except possibly in infancy, or in accelerating puberty, and relatively non-specific. It is not clear why odor release should be enhanced at the infertile time of menstruation, unless it overrules an infantile anxiety. The most likely true primer effects would be female>female or male>female—McClintock's chief example, if it is pheromonal, would be of the first kind: in this event male>female effects could also be sought with virtual certainty. The most likely of these, judging from mammalian form, are cycle modification or initiation (Lee and Boot, 1956), seen in mice, most herding animals (sheep, pigs) and among primates, in lemurs (Jolly, 1966); and acceleration of puberty (Vandenbergh, 1969). Human puberty certainly regressed to a late age during the height of Victorian purdah, and has since gotten steadily earlier (Tanner, 1962): this has occurred in both sexes and may well involve social factors—a pheromonal effect would be impossible to isolate. If it existed, it must presumably, in view of human family structure, depend on reinforcement by strangeness, and the presence of non-familial individuals. A pheromone effect triggered only during sex play or coitus could not easily be separated from the effects of direct stimulation, though there are such pheromones in primates (Michael and Saayman, 1967; Michael and Keverne, 1970), and human sex play has a large, though tabooed, orogenital component. Natural pheromone effects on fertility, implantation and the like (Bruce and Parkes, 1961) seem more remote in man, though they might be produced by synthetics and would be of great importance if found. The conceptuant and abortefacient effects of odor figured in medieval medical folklore, and musk and civet were among substances so credited.

A male>male effect cannot be ruled out. Its most likely form, on mammalian analogy, would be the release of aggression or submission, but distaste for foreign male odor seems to be reversible, for example in homosexuals (Ellis, 1905), and the fact that human male bonding is prominent could suggest that other interactions, such as puberty-timing in the male group, might be expected. The work of Kalogerakis (1963) implies a dominance effect between mature and immature males.

Chemical Substances

Beside the collection of considerable knowledge of insect pheromones, little has been done on mammalian smell components. The known candidates for pheromonal roles are those "self-selected" by man and used in perfumery (muskone, civetone, castoreum, and synthetics such as exaltolide), those derived from steroids and observed incidentally, such as boar taint, and a few special cases: cis-4-hydroxy-dodeca-6-enoic acid lactone in deer tarsal gland odor (Brownlee et al., 1969; Müller-Schwarze, 1969): response of some cat strains to valerianic acid and nepetalactone (Todd, 1962).

Michael's team (Curtis et al., 1971) has now identified the excitant substances for the male in the vaginal secretion of the female monkey and evoked a response with the synthetic mixture. The chief components are acetic, propionic, iso-butyric, n-butyric and iso-valeric acids. The same substances are present in the human vagina and contribute to its attractant odor, but do not make up its main subjective component, which is musky rather than acidic. The sexually excitant component of human genital odor is complex, involving both musk-like notes and odors akin to trimethylamine ("fishy") and is enhanced by alkaline fixatives. This "alkaline" odor component, which is not present in or compatible with the fatty-acid mixes effective in monkeys, is closely simulated both in certain plants recognized as sexual in folklore (Chenopodium vulvaria, Adoxa moschatellina) and in amine-rich hydrolized food extracts of yeasts ("Marmite") —the second of these has a fairly strong attractant effect on many cats. An alkaline component of the human male genital odor resembles another amine, 1,5 diaminopentane (cadaverine). Both these and the musky genital odor are enhanced by alkaline soaps and muted by acidic lotions. There may be a distinction here between subliminal releasers, which may well be fatty acids, and attractants, which may be cycloketonic, steroid or both. For humans, odors recognized as "sexual" are most commonly musk-like, though the axillary odor, and that of the feet (which in many animals are provided with tracking scent glands) are both excitant for many individuals and partly acidic. Odor fixed from foot apocrine glands may well play a part in the substitutional symbolism which erotizes the human foot.

Michael's findings apart, the substances of initial choice as probably releasers and possible primers in man are all musk odors (steroids, large-ring cycloketones and lactones) (Sink, 1967). The part played by 6, 8, and 10-carbon acids and lactones is unknown, but like the accessory non-steroid components of sweat, of smegma and of boar odor (Nitta and Ikai, 1953; Patterson, 1967, 1968) they probably have to do with detailed specificity. On this model the pheromone molecule is the key, and the subsidiary "notes," the wards adapting it to a particular biological lock, and possibly needed for reinforcement. Application of pheromones would probably require us to take account of both systems—the degree of functional specificity is likely to be as high in mammals as in insects, but more complex involving, for example, individual recognition. To this end the odor fingerprint approach of Dravnieks seems more promising than classical chemistry. Known musks might well serve as initial markers: the musky odor of human urine appears to be due to the -3-ol precursor of boar taint (Lederer, 1950) and nearly all 5α and 5β androstenones, as well as progesterone, have musky odor (Radt, 1959). The identity of mouse primer pheromones could be simply attacked by the methods of concentration used with insects—so far no article along these lines has appeared.

Sources of Pheromones

Many mammalian pheromones seem to be urinary, though specialized secretions are also common. Contact with urine plays little part in human relations, though it may be emphasized in paraphilias. More likely vehicles in man are the skin, including axillary and pubic apocrine glands and hair tufts, which resemble the deer's tarsal organ, and the smegma. The function of this secretion has been little studied, apart from its possible role in carcinogenesis. In the boar, its function seems to be to acquire odorous substances, either by secretion or fixation from preputial-sac urine, and "hold" them, possibly for conversion to an active state by bacterial action. Excision of the preputial glands reduces boar taint (Dutt et al., 1959) although the source of the steroid precursor is the gonad and adrenal (Sink, 1967). Humans lack the preputial sac, but male smegma contains a number of fixatives, including squalene (Sobel, 1949) and β-cholestanol esters, as well as other uncharacterized steroids (Kamat et al., 1960). Some odorants may be directly secreted, others fixed from urine or a partner. Odorous drugs, for example phenylethylhydrazine, are rapidly detectable in the human male genital odor. Deer musk is a direct preputial gland secretion and a fixative for secondary odors. Apocrine glands contribute to total body odor, but a smegma pheromone would be exposed precoitally with exposure of the glans, and would thus be analogous to the "response" substance in male moths; that is, a direct stimulus to receptivity. Odors fixed from a partner might also have a "playback" function, as in offspring labelling. Human female genital odor components have been studied by gas chromatography, but only in relation to the elimination of bacterial odor (Dravnieks et al., 1970).

The axillary secretion is a far more likely source of human social pheromones—possibly specialized, in view of the erect posture of man (Fitzherbert, 1959; Kloek, 1961). Odorous steroids such as progesterone are rapidly transferred to objects handled by a pregnant woman through the sweat generally, and the large human apocrine glands may be centers of such a function. The hair tufts probably serve as odor diffusers, as in deer, and may harbor activating bacteria (Shelley et al., 1953). Many substances are probably involved, including long-chain acids and lactones. Caproic, caprylic and capric acids were named from their "hircine" odor. Research in this field has been largely limited to deodorants and to identification of mosquito attractants in sweat (Skinner et al., 1965; Dravnieks et al., 1968). The peculiar odor of schizophrenics' sweat has been traced to trans-3-methyl hexanoic acid (Smith et al., 1969)—its significance is unknown.

There is a characteristic, powerful and pleasant axillary odor emitted only by women—some of them at all times, so that their presence in a room can be recognized, and others only occasionally. This odor, which resembles cumarone, appears to be unrelated to sexual excitement, but is itself attractant. It does not appear to be produced by males.

Apocrine sweat is almost wholly responsible for the normal odor of the clean human body, which differs markedly not only between "races" but between complexions within a polytypic population ("saucy and sometimes tiring in brunettes and black-haired women, sharp and fierce in redheads, it is heady and pervasive in blondes like the 'nose' of some flowery wines: you could almost say that it fits exactly with their manner of using the lips in kissing: firmer and more possessive in brunettes, more personal perhaps in blondes"—J. K. Huysmans Croquis parisiens 1880). Such literary descriptions refer to the female/male modality, but medieval authorities discriminate also the odor of chastity in both sexes (resembling ionone) and that of unchastity (resembling boiling starch). The odor of apocrine sweat appears to be released by bacterial action at the skin surface. That it changes with sexual excitement is a matter of common experience. Both in smegma and in apocrine hairtufts, bacteria may be true functional symbionts upon whose action odor release depends.

Prostaglandins, finally, may serve as non-olfactory pheromones. They are secreted in high concentrations in semen, and may stimulate uterine contractions which aid sperm transportation (H. A. Bern, personal communication, U.C., Berkeley).

A model of possible human pheromone effects can be plausibly constructed. The responsible substances are likely to occur in apocrine sweat and in smegma. They are likely to include odorous steroids, large-ring ketones, or other substanes perceived as musk-like. Accessory odors probably determine behavioral specificity rather than direct physiological action. Primer effects are most likely to be seen in the female; female-male effects may be limited to attraction, erection and so on and male-male effects may include dominance and attraction (bonding).

Odors fixed from a receptive partner may serve a "play-back" function. Reinforcement by strangeness may occur. There may be an extensive biology of imprinting and so on by odor in infant-parent and child-parent relations, which later undergoes repression or modification. Releaser and primer effects probably depend on the same materials, and may include substances fixed from urine, semen, or the sexual secretions of the other sex by smegma. The existence of primer effects in humans is unproven but likely. Odor fingerprinting and gas chromatography render the testing of these hypotheses immediately practicable.

The complexity of the "override" in human sexual behavior is such that, as in lemurs, menstrual synchrony and the like might well be subject to a mixed stimulus involving both pheromones and visual or social interaction. What strikes the biologist is that humans seem to possess a range of organs which we assume to be "vestigial" or non-functional, but which if we saw them in lower mammals, we should recognize as mediating odor exchanges. They include strategically placed hairtufts associated with apocrine glands; and that ethnographically persecuted appendage the foreskin, which permits the accumulation of a powerful fixative and brings it into contact with traces of urine, vaginal secretion and semen.

Platyrrhine monkeys use the sternal apocrine gland, homologous to our axilla, to mark out territory, and size is a measure of male dominance. The human tendency to attack and remove both body hairs and the prepuce as unesthetic may conceivably reflect an unconscious awareness of a biological association which we have missed at the conscious level. No biologist could now rule out, for certain, the possibility that these amputative practices have behavioral effects. At least, the belief that developed organs such as the appendix and tonsil "do nothing" and can be cut off without physiological effect is a naive one belonging to the last century.

We may be in for another shock. The time may be at hand when one can no longer tell an Alitalia plane by the fact that it has hair under its wings, and when deodorants, intimate and otherwise, rate with environmental pollution, as they already do among the sexually experienced. The notion of pheromonal influences on Man has often been mooted. It is still highly speculative, but could be important for medicine and psychiatry. We may live to see "odor therapy" move out of the realm of fringe medicine, into a field with wider implications, some beneficial, some frankly disquieting. The extreme economy of

the effect compared with the use of systemic hormones (some pheromones in insects operate at the single-molecule level) makes it well
worth examination in a culture which urgently needs all the control
over its reproductive processes that it can get.

References

Amoore, J. E. and J. Venstrom (1966) Sensory analysis of odor qualities in terms of the stereochemical theory. J. Food Sci. 31:118-128.

Bieber, I. (1959) Olfaction in sexual development and adult sexual
organisation. Am. J. Psychotherap. 13:851-859.

Brill, A. A. (1932) The sense of smell in the neuroses and psychoses.
Psychoanalytic Qu. 1:7-42.

Brooksbank, B. W. L. and G. A. D. Hazelwood (1950) The nature of
pregnanediol-like glucoside. Biochem. J. 47:36-43.

Brownlee, R. G., R. M. Silverstein, D. Müller-Schwarze and A. G.
Singer (1969) Identification, isolation and function of the male tarsal
scent in blacktailed deer. Nature (London) 221:284-285.

Bruce. A. M. and A. S. Parkes (1961) An olfactory block to implantation in mice. J. Reprod. Fert. 2:195-196.

Curtis, R. J., J. A. Ballantine, E. B. Keverne, R. W. Bonsall, and R. P.
Michael (1971) Identification of primate sexual pheromones and the
properties of synthetic attractants. Nature (London) 232:396-398.

Daly, C. D. and R. S. White (1930) Psychic reactions to olfactory
stimuli. Brit. J. Med. Psychol. 10:70-87.

Dravnieks, A., B. K. Krotoszynski, W. E. Lieb and E. J. Jungermann
(1968) Influence of an antibacterial soap on various effluents from
axillae. J. Soc. Cosmet. Chem. 19:611-612.

Dravnieks, A. and B. K. Krotoszynski (1970) Detection and identification of chemical signatures. U.S. Sci. Tech. Bull. Info. 1967 AD/691738.

Dravnieks, A., B. K. Krotoszynski, L. Keith and I. M. Bush (1970)
Odor threshold and gas-chromatographic assays of vaginal odors:
changes with nitrofurazone treatment. J. Pharm. Sci. 59:495-501.

Dutt, R. H., E. C. Simpson, J. C. Christian and C. E. Barnhardt (1959)
Identification of preputial glands as the site of production of sexual
odor in the boar. J. Anim. Sci. 18:1557-1558.

Ellis, H. (1905) Sexual Selection in Man. V. 4 (Davis, N.Y.).

Fitzherbert, J. (1959) Scent and the sexual object. Brit. J. Med. Psychol. 32:806-809.

Gleeson, K. K. and J. H. Reynierse (1969) The behavioral significance
of pheromones in primates. Psychol. Bull. 71:58-73.

Griffiths, N. M. and R. L. S. Patterson (1970) Human olfactory responses to 5α-androst-16-en-3-one, principal component of boar taint.
J. Sci. Food Agr. 21:4-6.

Groddeck, G. (1925) The Unknown Self (Daniel, London).

Jolly, A. (1966) Lemur Behavior (Chicago Univ. Press).

Kalogerakis, M. G. (1963) The role of olfaction in sexual development. Psychosom. Med. 25:420-432.

Kamat, V. N., T. B. Panse and V. R. Khanolkar (1960) Constituents of human smegma. Proc. Indian Acad. Sci. B. 52:1-8.

Kligman, A. M. and N. Shehadeh (1964) Pubic apocrine glands and odor. Arch. Dermatol. 89:461-463.

Kloek, J. (1961) The smell of some steroid sex hormones and their metabolites. Folia Psychiat. Neurol. Neurochir. Neer. 64:309-344.

Lederer, E. (1950) Odeurs et parfums des animaux. Fortschr. Chem. Org. Naturst. 6:87-153.

Lee, S. van der and Boot, L. M. (1956) Spontaneous pseudo-pregnancy in mice II. Acta Physiol. Pharmacol. Neer. 5:213-215.

Le Magnen, J. (1952) Les phénomènes olfactosexuels chez l'Homme. Arch. Sci. Physiol. 6:125-160.

McClintock, M. K. (1971) Menstrual synchrony and suppression. Nature (London) 299:244-245.

Michael, R. P. and E. B. Keverne (1970) Primate sex pheromones of vaginal origin. Nature (London). 255:84-85.

Michael, R. P. and G. Saayman (1967) Sexual performance index of male Rhesus monkeys. Nature (London). 214:425-626.

Müller-Schwarze, D. (1969) Complexity and relative specificity of a mammalian pheromone. Nature (London). 223:525-526.

Nitta, H. and H. Ikai (1953) Studies on the body odor. I. Separation of the lower fatty acids of the cutaneous excretion by paper chromatography. Nagoya Med. J. 1:217-224.

Patterson, R. L. S. (1967) A possible contribution of phenolic components to boar odor. J. Sci. Food Agr. 18:8-10.

Patterson, R. L. S. (1968) 5α-androst-16-en-3-one: Compound responsible for taint in boar fat. J. Sci. Food Agr. 19:31-38.

Radt, F., ed. (1959) Elseviers Ency. Org. Chem. Series III, 4, Suppl. 23955 seq. (Springer, Berlin).

Shelley, W. B., H. J. Harley and A. C. Nichols (1953) Axillary odor: an experimental study of the role of bacteria, apocrine sweat and deodorants. Arch. Dermatol. Syph. N.Y. 68:430-446.

Sink. J. D. (1967) Theoretical aspects of sex odor in swine. J. Theor. Biol. 17, 174-180.

Skinner, W. H., H. Tong, T. Pearson, W. Strauss and H. Maibach (1965) Human sweat components attractive to mosquitoes. Nature (London). 207:261-262.

Smith, K., G. F. Thompson and H. D. Koster (1969) Sweat in schizophrenic patients: identification of the odorous substance. Science 166:398-399.

Sobel, H. (1949) Squalene in sebum and sebum-like materials. J. Invest. Dermatol. 13:333-338.

Tanner, J. M. (1962) Growth at Adolescence (Blackwell, Oxford).

Todd, N. B. (1962) Inheritance of the catnip response in domestic cats. J. Hered. 63:54-56.

Vandenbergh, J. G. (1969) Effect of the presence of a male on sexual maturation in female mice. Endocrinology 84:658-660.

Vierling, J. S. and J. Rock (1967) Variation in olfactory sensitivity to exaltolide during the menstrual cycle. J. Appl. Physiol. 22:311-315.

Welch, L. and R. F. Hayes (1957) Elements in conditioning of normal and pathological human behaviour. J. Genet. Psychol. 91:263-293.

Whissell-Buechy, D. and J. E. Amoore (1973) Odor-blindness to musk. Nature (London) 242:271-273.

Wiener, H. (1966) External chemical messengers: I. Emission and reception in man. N.Y. State J. Med. 66:3153-3170.

Wiener, H. (1967a) External chemical messengers: 2. Natural history of schizophrenia. N.Y. State J. Med. 67:1144-1165.

Wiener, H. (1967b) External chemical messengers: 3. Mind and body in schizophrenia. N.Y. State J. Med. 67:1287-1310.

Wilson, E. O. (1963) Pheromones. Sci. Am. 208:100-114.

The Dwarf in the Middle

"Mathematics is the art of describing the same thing in
different language"—
Bertrand Russell

Modern neurology is beginning for the first time to address what must be the oddest as well as the most familiar of human characteristics—one so familiar that psychology, and all Western science, takes it for granted. This is the characteristic of our world view which goes by the infelicitous name of "homuncular I-ness"—the sensation, or more accurately the conviction, that there is "a little man inside" who initiates the actions of thinking, willing, and the like.

We are all so accustomed to this sensation that we take it for granted: if we tell a person to close his eyes and draw the E on his forehead, the subject will commonly read it as the figure 3—he "sees" it from behind. The positional sense of identity is a natural concomitant of binocular forward vision—a rabbit, with 360° visual field, would probably experience himself, if he were a discursive rabbit, more like· the central point of a circular radar scan.

Self-awareness of this kind has obvious practical implications, but it also has major significance for the Western tradition of science. This tradition, wherever it has spread, is based on the concept of an objective, external universe, which is consistent in its behavior, and can therefore be studied experimentally—its claim to objective reality rests on the fact that it is "not-I." This definition runs into trouble in disciplines like psychiatry when it addresses brain processes—are these to be regarded as part of "I" or as part of the environment? But for ordinary purposes the model holds and the intuitive view works. Descartes, in attempting to prove that *something* can be assumed to be real, started with the proposition "I must be real, because I am doing the thinking."

Technology has a way of turning philosophical conundrums into practical issues. With the growth of computer science, the problem of "I-ness" has proved no exception. The question has been asked, both by science fiction writers and by engineers, whether, if a mechanical thinking-system were to approach the complexity of a human brain, it too would develop self-awareness. Our sense of "I", which is basically a sense of ourselves as a focus distinct from everything else, which we call "the objective world", is not present in early childhood: a small baby appears to have difficulty in distinguishing his body at least, and quite possibly his "I-ness", from external objects. Accordingly it appears to be in part a learned mode of experiencing, and to acquire it a computer might have to have the equivalent of a human infancy, childhood and individuation. More to the point, existing computers have no need of individual "identity" because they are programmed to extend, and report to, the "I" of the programmer—for example, they are programmed to do mathematics intelligible to an abstracting mathematician and act as if they were mathematicians. But a computer designed to explore alternatives and objectivize when appropriate might quite possibly develop an internal device very like our sense of abstracted viewpoint.

A better way of putting the problem is to ask what could make a system objectivize itself. Put like this, it is a problem in systems theory, and some interesting answers are beginning to appear. Indian readers may be particularly interested in these because, unlike Western philosophy, the Indian tradition has always tended to treat I-ness as an illusory or at least an optional way of viewing self and not-self. Western psychologists and systems theorists coming fresh to the problem are beginning to find that there is a longstanding Sanskrit vocabulary to cover most of the matters under discussion—*ahamkara* for "homuncular I-ness" and *tat,* "THAT", for the non-I. By developing a very sophisticated technology of introspection, much Indian philosophy long since arrived at the conviction that both the experienced "I" *and* the picture which "I" have of the objective world are virtual or illusory. This conviction is based on the fact that there are states of mind, inducible by practice, occurring spontaneously, or—both in Vedic times and more recently in the West—facilitated by the use of drugs, in which "I-ness" is suppressed without the cessation of perception, and perceiver and perceived are experienced as non-different. These so-called oceanic experiences have been an important source of religious and philosophical insight precisely because they demonstrate experimentally that the objective-subjective distinction is an optional way of experiencing "reality"—the one to which empirical science is comitted because of its practical convenience, but not the only justifiable way.

How could a system be made to experience itself? There seem to be two plausible models, not necessarily mutually exclusive. Much recent work has been done on the differences between the logical-verbal mode of treating our experiential input, chiefly localized in the dominant hemisphere of the brain, and the Gestalt or pattern-seeing mode, which is nondiscursive, holistic, not verbally logical, and largely a function of the nondominant hemisphere (the localization is not rigid, as split-brain experiments show, but there do appear to be two distinct types of input-processing going on during normal experience). Now if we were to construct a perceiving "computer" in which such a two-channel method of analysis was incorporated, it is virtually certain that the two channels would have different time constants. If the two were to be compared, it would be necessary to divide the functioning of the faster into "bits" and introduce a time-delay network. The possibility exists that the odd experience which we call "identity"—the central reference-point, as it were, to which analyzed input is reported—is in fact an ongoing déjà-vu between two scanning processes, one of which, because of the difference in time constant, is able to monitor the activity of the other. This is precisely the model of the "two birds of like feather" in the Upanishadic parable, one of which feeds (experiences) while the other perceives and watches.

Some confirmation of such a model for "I"-ness comes from the fact that if subjects watch themselves in a "delaying mirror" (closed-circuit television with an 0.5-0.25 sec delay), some people experience an odd illusion of multiple or dual identity, rather as playback of speech interferes with its fluency. It also focusses experimental attention on drugs and traditional meditative exercises which interfere with the sense of I-ness and induce oceanic experience. Intense meditation on the process itself and on the *nature* of I-ness is one of these—flooding, or by contrast withdrawal, of sensory input is another.

In the oceanic experience, not only does the subject cease to experience the objective self as distinct from what is not-self but the experience is accompanied by powerful sensations of nondiscursive knowledge, wholeness, rightness and identity with the entire structure of the world. This might mean simply that the verbalizing limb of the "bridge" has been silenced, so that pattern alone is perceived, or that the time-lag has somehow been removed (*samādhi* could be translated not only as oceanic experience, but also as "making equal"). A different model may perhaps throw more light on this.

Karl Pribram at Stanford has recently suggested that the brain functions not like a computer but like a hologram. A hologram is a photo-record of the interference-fringes produced by wave-fronts reflected at a given wavelength from an array. When viewed in ordinary light it appears as a blur, but when scanned with the coherent beam of a laser, solid objects appear and can be made to rotate or to move relative to each other by tilting the hologram. Another property of a hologram is that if it is cut up and a small portion is scanned, the whole scene appears, though at a decreasing level of definition—in other words, all parts of the hologram contain all of the information contained in the whole.

On this model, what we normally experience could be the scanned state of the interference-pattern generated in the brain by sensory inputs and by its own activity. In an oceanic or "I-less" mode of perception, the scan would be shut off, and what is intuited would then be the interference-pattern itself. Conventional attempts to represent the oceanic vision as "music of the spheres," a many-petalled lotus, or a receding structure of superimposed triangles, bear some resemblance to, or analogy with, interference patterns, and all such subjective records stress the continuation and heightening of perception, but with the sense of external viewpoint suppressed.

Our only contact with a "real" world is by way of the sensory inputs we receive from it, and the conceptual and classifying processes which go on in the brain. If both of these are expressed in some form of interference pattern, oceanic states may represent a trick by which this pattern is monitored without being interpreted: in this case the processes connected with our sense of the objective would be of a piece with the rest of the hologram, and the positional "I" would be seen as containing the information of the whole, like any other subdivided hologram. Switch on the scan again and separate objects and concepts would once more be seen as separate.

All of this speculation was initially long on creative theory and very short on experimental fact—before we commit ourselves to a "holographic model" for the brain, there are some awkward questions to ask; not least the nature of the waves of electrical activity which produce the hypothetical interference-pattern: presumably they represent the sum-and-difference of phase relations between the activity of different synapses. Since it is now possible to record brain activity, not as waves, but as a power-spectrum which can be scanned like a hologram, using the circuitry developed for side-looking radar, Pribram's model should be investigable.

This is now proving to be the case. Pribram (1974, 1979) cites a whole range of neuropsychological studies on image formation to support the active role played by brain mechanisms in putting together "wholes" out of sensory inputs by a combination of computational and optical-type information processes. The momentary states set up in the course of this processing activity closely resemble those of image-constructing devices—in other words, they are holographic. The same applies to memory: rules are stored as in a computer, but images are retrieved from a holographic "deep structure." Pribram's own work has shown that the anatomic localization of motor functions in the cortex functions as an "array" on which environmental invariances are displayed. One interesting confirmation of this comes from the discrepancy between two experiments in which kittens were raised in a striped environment. In one case, conducted by Blakemore in 1974, the stripes were painted on the walls of the cylinder in which the animals were raised—these kittens were thereafter unable to follow the movement of a bar traveling at right angles to the direction of the stripes. Hirsch and Spinelli, in Pribram's laboratory, raised kittens in striped goggles, and found no change in their behavior as a result. It follows from this that to affect behavior the constant input had to remain invariant across transformations produced by head and eye movements—which is what one would expect of a holographic rather than a "perceptual" mode of processing.

More recent experimental evidence is even more specific (Pribram 1974, 1979). What started as a "powerful metaphor" to account for the mathematics of perception has been convincingly demonstrated to operate in fact, at least over the area of image encoding in the cortex. It needs to be pointed out to nonbiological as well as to philosophical readers that nobody has proposed that *all* brain systems are holographic. Besides the apparatus of imaging, the spatial representation of inputs, and their processing in memory and recognition, there must also be readout systems congruent with the creation of conventional or object-centered perception, including language, which is largely the process of giving names to the objects so created. Brain holography is best seen as a department of brain function, like the memory bank in a computer, but more versatile and fundamental than this. A dichotomy between encoding as image and readout as object or verbalization aptly fits the two-channel model for identity processes: identity in this view goes with the focussed or object-forming mode present in the sense organs (quintessentially the eye, where an optical image is formed as in a camera). The two realities, which one might call optical and holographic realities, require different time-constants because one is synoptic while the other involves reduction into "bits", so that the identification of I-ness with the predominance of optical reality in everyday experience is practical, not confined to philosophical argument over how far the whole idea of transcendental identity in objects is a position artefact arising from the human experience of personal identity.

Even more important than the model, however, is the refocussing of our attention on just how far positional identity as a normal mode of experience biases our conception of the world. Science always has a hard time transcending common sense intuitions, of which this must be by far the most compelling, far less accessible to correction or additional intuition than the "flat earth." The more we think about and investigate neuropsychological processes, the more evident it becomes that the kind of structure which we see as being objective depends on the system which is doing the seeing as much as on what is there to be seen. The "real" might be grossly counterintuitive—in collapsing time, for example, or not containing cause-effect—and if it were it could not, with conventional human intellectual equipment, be experienced, though it could be and is being inferred. At the intuitive level, it spite of particle physics, our intuitive vision still has to work in terms of discrete objects. Mathematics is a partial recourse, because we can appeal to our holographic equipment to identify an esthetic "rightness," but the actual pattern, like the answer to a *koan,* can only be apprehended in an oblique, and hence traditionally unsatisfactory, way.

The actual material of scientific discourse obviously represents a selective mode of seeing, but the teaching is that investigation can inherently dissolve fundamental illusions. This was true enough of the flat earth, but we still do not empathize the inverted posture of Australians. In spite of Heisenberg and his own laboratory findings, the most sophisticated physicist, while knowing that my table and my typewriter are not "things" but repercussions of local accumulations of energy, is in no better posture than a savage to *see* them in that light. The dissolution of self-evident parts of experience such as time and causality cannot be directly empathized in a mode compatible with daily activity, though in doing science it may have, like the square root of –1, to be taken as given.

Mathematics has been the life-preserver of physics in this area because creative mathematicians are accustomed to this sort of thing. They have found a mode in the equipment which makes it possible to visualize, say, Lobaschevskian space, without trying to render it into conventional experience, except by way of rough diagrams, rather as a mediaeval artist indicates that a person is a saint by depicting him with light coming out of his head.

None of this is a problem in interpreting a holographic brain model. The mathematics are conventional, and the brain is a physical object from which electrical and other measurements can be taken. It gets to be relevant because of the sharp reminder it gives us of the artefactual character of most of our habitual modes of thinking; we see things as things, but our brain, for its own purposes, does not.

The uncertainty principle originally sets forth the incompatibility between measurements which fundamentally interfere with one another. The existence of a heavily-programmed, adaptive and prosaic sense of reality and of I-ness presents a second, Goedelian type of uncertainty principle, connected with the problem of using one and the same brain to generate the motivated, investigating I, to criticize the intuitive, and to work out its own manner of working.

Over a large part of practical science, the intuitive model has worked and continues to work—for these purposes argument as to how far our perceptions of, say, fossils, influenza viruses or comets are "real" is merely diversionary—like a denial that terrestrial surfaces are flat when one is laying tiles. Physics, which is the area in which the intuitive model has run out the soonest, is to some extent buffered by being able to rely on mathematics to make counter-intuitive thinking possible. But even here mathematical treatment only postpones a philosophical crunch. We are running the human ideational system, if not close to its limits, at least in a highly unusual mode; the method of processing in the system we are using becomes increasingly important, and one part of that system is the intuitive Cartesian "I" which cogitates and therefore is.

Pribram's model of brain process as hologram might make one look for other holographic-type structures: what about "objective reality" itself? This has moved from hard objects to aggregations of hard atoms, then to aggregations of energy, and finally to the behavior of loci in space-time. This kind of speculation well illustrates the neurological bind. It might be that the brain is holographic. It might be that the mathematics of holograms have heuristic value when applied, for example, to particle physics. Suppose they do—does that mean that "the universe is a hologram" in some fundamental sense, or simply that if one projects a different neural model involved in the sorting processes in our own heads, one gets a different paradigm for what is "real"?

Science has advanced as a practical activity by sensibly ignoring this kind of speculation for as long as possible—its potential as a philosophical quagmire leading to mystification is enormous. But with continued technical successes, the hard ground seems to be running out. It did so, in fact, some time ago in physics: in Heisenberg's words "the conception of objective reality has evaporated into a mathematics that no longer represents the behavior of elementary particles, but rather our knowledge of this behavior." "There is no cause or effect in nature: nature simply *is*: recurrence of like cases exists but in the abstraction we perform for the purpose of mentally reproducing facts" (Mach). In this new scientific world, "nature" consists of arrays—which may for all we know be infinite in number—and from this "interference pattern" our sensorium pulls out structures to fit itself. Phenomena, which are our only mode of contact with this multifarious "nature," are exactly what the name says, appearings, in which structure has been selectively added. Moreover, in some cases ("time" and "space" are probable instances) what look like phenomena turn out to be structures connected with our conviction of positional identity and the fact that, if it depends for operation on a delay network, time processes cannot be run backwards.

Nobody is, of course, suggesting that the "array" existing in nature contains no real phenomena which can be abstracted as space and time—only that the human habit of abstracting them greatly affects the formalisms we use. We have a computing system which is like that.

One way to look at it is to put ourselves in the shoes of my demon friend, Gezumpstein. Gezumpstein is a highly intelligent demon who differs from human mathematicians in having no sense of positional or temporal identity. Can we figure out how Gezumpstein's mathematics would look? Gezumpstein was never a baby and did not learn to count fingers, but he has been obliged to invent numerals as an algebraic convenience. He comprehends the content of expressions in the form:

$$a + b = c$$

but since he does not experience the naive or nonmathematical overtones of algebra, he has absolutely no incentive to write them like that. In other words, his mathematical perception owed nothing to practical experiences that a spatially separated a and b when put in one place amount to c, or that first there were a and b and these generated a c, both of which would be quite alien to his way of seeing. Instead, Gezumpstein experiences addition directly in the form that the set of c's is completed by the set of a's and the set of b's. Gezumpstein reads Feynman diagrams without any time arrow and, anticipating Bolzmann intuitively, without any idea of the "identity" of particles, since identity is not part of his world. Moreover, unlike us, he is not tied to either-or choices when confronted with two options—A and not-A—because unlike us, he can see coherent superpositions.

Suppose that in some way Gezumpstein becomes aware of a chess game. Being an intuitive mathematician, he at once sees that it is a meaningful gestalt, but for him it is made up of mathematical quantities ("moves") made up in turn of peculiar quanta ("squares"). He is intrigued by this intuition of structure. He finds that he can apply a sequential analysis (though he does not call it that) in the form

if (A)...then (B)

and can thereby codify these peculiar abstractions (his vocabulary, of course, includes neither "then" nor "because"). He also does not distinguish, e.g., individual pawns as having identities. In Gezumpstein's case, skullsplitting counterintuitive thinking leads him to postulate a field ("space") in which moves can be depicted, though neither he nor the most erudite of his fellow-demons can visualize such a thing. He suspects that there is a second classification ("time") but cannot pin it down. One limit of the pattern, he knows, is the linear arrangement in "space" of all of the pieces facing each other and the other is a constellation of moves involving the king, but how to express the relationship defeats him.

Gezumpstein is short on arithmetic and equations, long on field theory and topology, though his "surfaces" are wholly abstract, not models. Forces when he observes them look to him uncommonly like "things", but "things" in our Democritean sense are a very hard notion and he does not postulate them. Since his mathematics is wholly nonsequentially presented, it cannot be typed-in on a moving tape and does not consist of a sequence of operations. It "contains neither cause nor effect, it just is." So Gezumpstein's "space" and "time" if he finally postulates them are mathematical conveniences designed to vary his intuitive inclusivism, and the idea of causality, if he postulates that, a very upsetting systems break which threatens his whole intuitive way-of-seeing.

The interesting part about Gezumpstein is that his world, like Flatland, reveals some of our built-in preconceptive ways of dealing with data. Both we and he would get to the same place, but by very different routes.

The point of the exercise involved in creating Gezumpstein is to see how a world view would look if it were not based on the conceptualizations which inhere in positional I-ness. Most of the conventions involved in Einsteinian space-time are complex attempts to square observation with the shape given to phenomena by a Cartesian I who is doing the observing, and to whom phenomena appear. Two interesting psychiatric points arise from this. One is that because visualized models *have* to be identity-regarding (translated, that is, into formalisms which a time-and-space-positional I can visualize) the revolution involved in quantum physics has had absolutely no impact on the day-to-day world view even of people who work with it: unlike the discoverers of the Copernican and Newtonian world they experience no reordering of consciousness—they say, "How intensely interesting" and go home to dinner. Aside from occultists who rub their hands at the idea that there may be other worlds, fourth dimensions and so on to vindicate their preconceptions, modern physics has had no religious and rather little philosophical impact. If it could somehow be popularly empathized, it would be a blockbuster.

The second is that if there are available Gezumpstein-like states of mind in which such complex models, instead of being computed, are directly perceived, as we normally perceive in terms of conventional space and conventional time, they might "do the trick"—not only in providing a new mathematical and scientific resource, but in altering their possessors' world view as well. Now this is what "mystics" and other cultivators of oceanic states have always claimed. So far they have been uninterested in the physical universe and given to making the religious noises required by their particular tradition. Most have been far more moved by the components in the experiences they sought which led to feelings of one-ness (with God, with the Brahman) and which probably owe their attraction to emotions connected with the psychoanalytic stock-in-trade of human individuation. It would take a tough, rather than an analyzed, yogi to set these intoxicant psychedelia aside, and set about making the ineffable effable in terms of world models. Westernized yogis, when genuine and tough, still point out the difficulties of thinking about physics while in a state of samadhi—most bring back only a salutary experience of the condition-ality of conventional perception. A computer, with no Kleinian back-log, might do better—present computers neither do, nor are likely to, exhibit human I-ness because at present they are programmed to act like, and report to, a homuncularly oriented mathematician, who *provides* the Cartesian observer.

This need not be so. If we could infer how things would look to Ge-zumpstein we could program a system, holographic or otherwise, to think in Gezumpsteinian terms—to treat alternative events, for ex-ample, as both/and rather than either/or and handle divergent time-streams, rather as a chess computer rehearses all possible moves. If·it could choose all of them rather than the most probable, it would see the matrix of all chess games, not play a particular game. Gezump-stein, who thinks like this, has a problem making sense of chess be-cause he has a problem extracting the thread of play which corre-sponds to conventional perception. But we shall need some hard and inspirational math to copy him.

For a start, Gezumpstein's intellectual problems would be largely solved if he recognized that his intuitive "reality" differs from ours, or can be brought into line with ours, by the intervention of what amounts to a Fourier transformation: Gezumpstein is perceiving, by our standards, holographically. Our sensorium receives frequency-encoded input and, on Pribram's model, stores it by frequency-encoded engrams; but between the two focussing intervenes, and it is the focussed or de-transformed image which figures as our conven-tional or intuitive reality, complete with a representation in space-time and the visualization of discrete objects. This raises the interesting (and for some), disturbing probability that in giving philosophic defi-nitions of what is "real" and what is "phenomenal," Gezumpstein—who is not bugged in his perceptions by a positional I—is quite likely. to be right.

All "Western" non-Pythagorean thought prior to Heisenberg has tended to regard the conventional or intuitive "focussed" version ("middle-order reality") as in some way primary, even if it required relativistic correction, and its Fourier derivates as convenient mathe-matical transformations. It is just as possible, however, to regard Fourier patterns as the primary "objective reality" and the conventional world as a transform, produced by evolution because of the high convenience of space-time and causality in dealing practically with middle-order objects, and therefore adaptive. One thing which it generates is the convenient congruence of sensory impressions—by transforming to generate objects, we can usually assure that what we see we can also touch, if it is in the category of objects.

In support of this idea that our mode of seeing is a special case adaptive to things we might normally expect to see in unsophisticated conditions, one can point out that it works so well over the range from a grain of sand to a distant star that it produces no awkwardnesses— these arise only at the cosmic and the subatomic levels, when we are trying to make consistent sense not of direct perceptions but of inferences. It is in these areas, outside the range for which our particular sensorium was "made a-purpose" that paradoxes start to multiply. One advantage of a Gezumpstein-Fourier model for primary reality is that it does in fact deal with several troublesome paradoxes, ranging from the double-take between particulate and wave-mechanical models (the "Copenhagen solution") to some of the deficiencies of classical molecular biology and genetics in fully explaining morphogenesis—the type of problems, recently examined by Goodwin by way of Laplacian transformations, which drove biologists like Driesch into neovitalism.

There is, moreover, a steady revival in physics of interference models on other grounds, in the work of Wheeler and Bohm (1971, 1973) for example. This is not a new idea: for Hindu philosophy, field-type reality is Brahman and the intuitive or focussed transform is māya, the type of perception which generates space-time and discrete objects. But it is new as a heuristic hypothesis, at least since Pythagoras generalized that "reality" was analogous to music in its structure. In the flush of enthusiasm it has of course to be pointed out that holographic models for brain imaging, morphogenesis and particle physics resemble the close similarity of the curves for the growth of pumpkins, bacterial populations, and the gross national product of Ruritania. They may represent either analogy or homology, or (in the case of holographic representations) the direct effects of brain mechanisms on human conceptualization. This is a difficult one. Pribram's holographic brain model, despite some vigorous dissent from reputable physiologists, looks evidentially very plausible. We have no mechanism of any description, even among computers, which can address reality (whatever that is) without the intervention somewhere along the line of a human brain—in fact, *without* a human brain there are philosophical problems in giving a meaning to the word "reality" and even to the word "meaning". There are the beginnings here of a Catch 22 situation. However, the assignment of experimental science is basically to get around and behind precisely this dependence of concepts on the apparatus which does the conceptualizing, and the same brain has proved a versatile instrument for this kind of low cunning. It should be possible to aim experiments to pick up the counter-intuitive in this area as in others. Particle physics, where middle-order reality simply falls apart, is a good place to start. In conventional "reality", transfer of properties from one apparent entity to another is usually prohibited; action at a distance is worrying, as it was to both Newton and Einstein, and calls for a cumbersome construction which then remains around as a challenge to produce mathematical syntheses between postulated forces. In the transform it presents no problems. By translational invariance, any change is represented in all parts of the field, and vehicular particles—gluons and other kinds of boson—may not be required (Capra, 1978). Nobody is bothered if virtual particles behave as if they were "real" particles, since all particles are on this view virtual.

This is not the place to expound on the steady growth of field theories in the area of quantum physics—they have recently been surveyed by Nash (1978). The point is that even strictly mathematical models like the Weinberg-Salam unified field theory, which aims at a reductionist model for the observed forces, are in a sense as much covertly concerned with brain physiology as with attributes of nature: whether a theory is unified or includes systems breaks and multiplication of entities depends on properties of the processing system. Middle-order reality is such a practical device for unification—it involves the generation of conceptual "objects" relevant to ordinary living, on which the senses can, as it were, converge operationally. It therefore defines *a* reality, the object of which is practical. Pre-Einsteinian physics did the same. Now, however, our practicalities are changing—there is nothing unpractical about quarks or tachyons, since our comprehension of them may very well have practical spinoffs. This is the difference between our scientific pragmatism and the more self-indulgent-looking exercises of Hindu and Buddhist nonobjectivizing philosophy, which quite frankly aim at a spiritual quality of comprehension and are not specially interested in the regularities of *māya* or middle-order reality—if it is virtual or illusory, why bother about it? Physicists, however, seem to be discovering these models, aimed in a very different direction, with glee. Starting from the work of Chew at the Lawrence Berkeley Laboratory on S-matrix theory, Capra (1975) has pointed out the likeness between such concepts of "bootstrapping" and the Taoist intuition of a "grain" in nature.

Gezumpsteinian algebra, or what has equally jocularly been called topsicology (for structures which are field-determined and accordingly appear to "just grow") has a further use as a heuristic tool not in physics but in biology. Organisms are real-time and middle-order-reality substrates, but both their phylogeny and the epigenetic development were constantly fought over by philosophically-inclined biologists from Cuvier on. Most of the energy of modern hard-nosed science has had to be devoted to fighting off, successively, naive creationism and neovitalism. Neither is dead, but molecular genetics did at one time appear to have done the reductionist trick, both in evolutionary theory and in embryology.

This is no longer strictly true. For a start, in embryogenesis, genes appear to be far more the providers of available materials than the generators of developmental fields, leaving the big question, "What exactly determines that, of cells having identical genetic structure, some produce an eye and others a toenail?" In speciation, Darwinian selectionist models are the models of choice, but they present some awkward problems calling for acts of faith, recourse to indirect selection and the like, which we dutifully make (so as not to give comfort to people who want to fell us with Genesis ch. 1), but which creak. Maynard Smith's acrostic paradox—how to effect by selection the transition from one encoded character to another without going through a disadaptive or nonsense combination—is the least of these.

It is interesting, purely as an intellectual exercise, to substitute the Gezumpsteinian model. This, in regard to speciation, involves abandoning the historical and Linnean tree-shaped grids on which phylogeny is now usually depicted and applying S-matrix formalisms. Analogies now appear between channeling in microphysics and canalization in Waddington's sense. Both are probabilistic: the nodes are in one case read as particles and in the other as species or in embryogenesis, as organs. In the last century, Lindley (1846) did indeed try to classify plants not in a Linnean tree but on a chessboard type of matrix, very like the periodic table; but the implications of this were missed. One consequence of the transformation is that the apparent quantum behavior of speciation is emphasized—"missing links" represent prohibited states.

This approach involves rewriting evolution (leaving out heredity-mechanisms for the moment) as if species were particles, rather as do simultaneous creationists, but with quite other consequences. An exactly similar transformation can be done in the Laplacian analysis of embryonic gradients. If the artificiality of these in terms of natural history leads to protest, that is only because we have analogized from everyday experience that the historical or genealogical model is ex *hypothesi* the most productive. We are big boys now, and do not need to reinforce ourselves against the risks of falling into biblical fundamentalism or supernatural vitalism: in other words, we can use two contradictory models as supplementary tools without intellectual risk, Euclid and Riemann, Newton and Einstein, with the habitual finding that if the models are well chosen both will prove of heuristic importance.

One need no more be a Hindu to treat objects as events or loci in an interdependent field than one needs to be Jewish to like rye bread: interestingly enough, Indian physicists have been too close to the Tradition to draw directly on it as a source of ideas in this area. The germs of field theory in Western thought may well have come there by way of Buddhist influences on Stoicism (Comfort, 1979), but Indian scientists are probably just as scared as most Westerners of the influence of "religion" on science. However, if a religion is a world view defining the relations of the experience of I-ness to a hypothetical That, scientific objectivism qualifies as one no less than does Hinduism or Buddhism.

We do not accordingly start from, or need, any soft generalizations about brain-as-microcosm: the brain-as-perceiving system model will do nicely and is more in line with critical analysis. Our brain need not be universe-shaped (though it may be) because our universe is bound to be brain-shaped. At the same time, once we start looking critically at the preconceptions generated by our experience of positional identity, we have to re-examine the instrument we are using. In the case of particles we have had to stop attributing transcendental identity to these hypothetical objects (Post, 1963). There is no way around the closed loop implicit in the *cogito,* awkward as it is; slap-happy excursions into pure mentalism which take the line that "mind is the only reality" will always run into the fact that if we are using a nervous system to think, that too is part of middle-order reality, and risk the conventional fate of objects which fly in ever-decreasing circles. There is still going to be a system break at the point where we have to explain how matter sets about thinking itself if it is virtual and a construct of our material sensorium.

This is something on which people like Sankara and Nagarjuna are either deliberately obscure, or led to take refuge in a kind of cosmic engram which stands behind I-ness and is the true dwarf in the middle. Labelling this as Brahman and then translating Brahman and māya as "God" and "illusion" rather than as field and phenomenal reality add further to the confusion, and fuel edifying rather than illuminating interpretations based on what *we* have traditionally attributed to God. Spinoza brought very much the same problem down on himself in the same way, and I risk doing so by treating objective science as a religion, which anthropologically it is. Nor are Hindus and Buddhists necessarily more consistent than we are: they talk traditionally about reincarnation (in linear time) and the unreality of time in the same doctrinal breath. Where esoterica might help us is not in being harder-nosed, but in acquiring direct experience of Gezumpstein's world. For this reason it is a perfectly serious comment that a systematic pursuit of "oceanic" perception, starting with traditional methods, might help us in intuiting how a thingless or holographic universe might look, never mind the materiality, middle-order-reality style, of our cortex.

For some time now, visualizations have not been much help in modern physics; it was far simpler, in Newtonian days, when they were. Unfortunately, the simple methods of producing I-less modes of perception are unreliable, but if physicists were able to take advantage of a Western, neurology-assisted version of more traditional yogas they might find them an invaluable aid to comprehension. It is one thing to dream up a "holographic" universe in terms of higher mathematics, and quite another to experience the conditionality of common sense perceptions such as causality or the linearity of time. One can imagine this kind of exercise going into the mathematics course for astrophysicists rather as marine biologists now routinely learn scuba diving. The results would be novel, however traditional the methods, because the cultures which developed them for religious purposes did not have the motivation to apply them, in the crass Western manner, to practical issues like atomic structure.

This kind of argument used to enrage traditional Hindus, rather as J.B.S. Haldane enraged biblical Christians by trying to compute how thick a breastbone an angel would need to support his wing muscles. As a matter of fact Haldane, a hardnosed rationalist and Marxist to boot, was one of the first Western biologists to listen attentively to what Hindu philosophers were saying. The practical implication of adopting their viewpoint and devoting serious attention to the experience of "I-ness" is that not only neurology but physics will turn its attention to our chief and our only indispensable scientific instrument, the human brain, and its odd assumption of observerhood. At this point Indian philosophers from Shankaracharya on could be pardoned for saying to the West, "So what else is new?" Western science in the objectivizing tradition has plugged away at its own sādhana (which is really the only basis on which it can be expected to listen to other people's insights) until it has reached the point at which it is obliged to devise techniques of analytic introspection directed at the human way-of-seeing. Indian philosophers have started with the human way-of-seeing and developed a sophisticated technology of introspective experiment, using the computer to monitor itself. In other words, each tradition got to the same concerns in its own way. I can imagine that just as some hard-line Western scientists will go on regarding Indian philosophers as poetic but unregenerate mystics, some Indian philosophers will see a neurology of I and That as one more Western attempt to de-sacralize experience and get everything down to a derivate of matter. If so, the progress of physics and of neurology will quite simply knock our heads together to our mutual benefit; heuristic science is a brisk purge for the sloppy, the theosophically-inclined or the fanciful in hypothesis-making, and the technology of introspection a sedative for simplistic bumptiousness, and it is this, rather than chatter about Western materialism and Eastern spirituality, which is next on the agenda. Western physics might benefit from a direct contact with traditional Hindu philosophy and empiricism derived by reading the Sanskrit literature, not by way of itinerant swamis who preach in mottos out of fortune cookies. A very interesting shift in our world view might result.

Bibliography

Bohm, D. Quantum theory as an indication of a new order in physics. Part A. The development of new orders as shown through the history of physics. Foundations of physics 1971 1:359-381.

Bohm, D. Quantum theory as an indication of a new order in physics. Part B. Implicate and explicate order in physical law. Foundations of physics, 1973.

Capra, F. The Tao of Physics. New York, Random House, 1975.

Capra, F. Quark physics without quarks: a review of recent developments in S-matrix theory. Lawrence Berkeley Laboratory USDE LBL-7596 (preprint) 1978.

Comfort, A. I and That: Notes on the Biology of Religion. New York, Crown Publrs., 1979.

Heisenberg, W. The representation of nature in contemporary physics. Daedalus 87:95-108, 1958.

Lindley, J. The Vegetable Kingdom. London, Bradbury and Evans, 1846.

Mach, E. In J.R. Newman: The world of mathematics. New York, Simon and Schuster, 1956, p. 1708.

Nash, C. Relativistic Quantum Fields. London, Academic Press, 1978.

Post, H. Individuality and physics. Listener, November 10, 1963.

Pribram, K. H., Nuwer, M. and Baron, R. The holographic hypothesis of memory structure in brain function and perception. In Atkinson, R.C., Krantz D.H., Luce R.C. and Suppes P.: Contemporary Developments in Mathematical Psychology. San Francisco, W.H. Freeman Co., 1974, pp. 416-467.

Pribram, K.H. Behaviorism, phenomenology and holism in psychology: a scientific analysis. J. soc. biol. Struct., 1979.

Religio Medici

Philosophy may in recent years have been a hobby for those doctors who had time for it, or who had retired from practice, but it has seldom had very much value on the wards or in the office. My own generation sat occasionally under teachers who recommended it as "broadening" (they presumably meant that it was part of a general education), but that breed is extinct. The modern medical student, however, is back in the situation which preceded the long period of 19th century scientism. Prior to that, student physicians did study philosophy occupationally, and doctors were among its busiest practitioners. What they meant by philosophy, however, was what we call experimental science—"natural philosophy"—not Kant, Wittgenstein and G.E. Moore. Although general science in the 18th century was not of great assistance to clinical work, it was obvious from the time of Francis Bacon on that one day it would be. Natural philosophy proceeded to multiply by simple fission—it passed through the principia which we learn in the premedical course and subdivided until it resembled the Mississippi Delta. Medical students, sailing chiefly on the streams called anatomy and physiology, and under time-pressure then as now, stopped looking through telescopes and reading any but clinical and pharmaceutical chemistry.

At the same time "philosophy"—the general theory of reality—got a divorce from "science" and retired to play word-games for which the man on the wards or in the operating room, having a fairly good grasp of the kind of realities he was obliged to handle, had very little time. The payoff of science, so evident in the Industrial Revolution, lagged in medicine. When Queen Victoria's husband died of typhoid, The Times described medicine as the withered arm of science. Then Pasteur and the early anesthesiologists started their raids on medicine from the field of chemistry, with the bacteriologists close on their heels, and after them Ehrlich and chemotherapy, the Curies and radiobiology, Gowland Hopkins and the new science of biochemistry. The Mississippi had put itself together again and was pouring over the head of the medical student: all of it complex, all of it relevant, all of it needed not only in answering multiple choice questions but in the actual practice of medicine and the acquisition of further knowledge.

Even mathematics is a required subject—we use statistical analysis to evaluate our clinical findings. No other discipline has had quite such a bath. (In no other discipline would it be reasonable to put papers on medical practice, psychoanthropology, psychobiology, and physics into a single book in the expectation that the audience will have some idea what one is talking about.)

Moreover, science and philosophy recently re-married—or if you prefer it, philosophy is now natural-philosophy again, because the post-Newtonian world view, Gezumpstein's world, depends on the results of physical experimentation, and the findings of physical experimentation indicate that what we find depends on the brain we use to categorize the results. Accordingly, the observations of those most philosophical of philosophers—the explorers of inner space—suddenly acquire a high degree of relevance to science itself.

Very fortunately, in most areas of medicine we are dealing with middle-order phenomena affecting cells, organs, organisms and organic molecules. The Gezumpsteinian model is active in advanced physics—it may, or may not, have relevances in biology. But, thank God, we do not need to bring quantum logic into internal medicine, or not yet, not for a long time (if ever). Our main reason for understanding it may be in finding ammunition to convince California patients that nothing so far observed can be used to validate astrology, pyramidology, or a general return to superstition as a substitute for proper health care. Their interest in meditation is another matter, as I will suggest further along.

There was a previous occasion in the history of natural philosophy when Gezumpsteinian and nonintuitive models of reality were seriously examined, but the examination was premature. Luckily for European science, we elected instead, about 1660, to take the course in Newtonian, mechanistic, middle-order fundamentals. The opposite choice occurred at the start of the 17th century, at the short-lived court of the Protestant King of Bohemia, and its luminaries were proto-Californians—numerologists, charismatics, alchemists (the forerunners of particle physics, these, who started too far up the scale of thermodynamic complexity, got no results, but spotted intuitively that there was a link between patterns of "reality" and human mental structures), Christian yogis—in fact everyone of whom the Roman Church disapproved and who disapproved of the Roman Church. It was a heady, uncritical, Californian brew, but its ideas attracted some of the leading minds of the day—not only John Dee the mystic and mathematician, but Leibnitz, Descartes and Newton himself. But the Bohemian Protestant monarchy fell after a year, the Gezumpsteinian speculators were scattered, or avoided the subject for fear of the Inquisition, and instead of the "invisible Rosicrucian College" which they planned, Elias Ashmole and his friends formed the visible and experimental Royal Society. Hard science won out—though Newton, Leibnitz and Descartes never lost their interest in the possibility of a second order of reality.

Much of what they surmised, which made poor sense to them, makes far better sense to us, with Heisenberg, Mach and Schroedinger under our belts, to say nothing of Carl Jung. It is still "background"— nobody needs to understand the world-models kicked around by David Bohm and John Wheeler to take out an appendix or to treat acute depression. In fact in psychiatry we are still fighting off a softheaded nonmedical model arising from the misunderstanding of psychoanalysis which would have reduced Freud to despair: his head was one of the hardest in medical history, and today he would have had primate ethology and neuropharmacology to keep him afloat.

The one area in which this new comprehension of the factitious character of middle-order reality impinges on medicine is in the area of our own and our patients' beliefs, because neither we nor they have caught up with it. The physicist's world is impossible to visualize, and although yogis have visualized the Gezumpsteinian position for several thousand years we are not yogis and our patients do not come from a tradition which produces them. Yogis took the trouble they did because the crunch of transcending middle-order constructs is unsustainable by ordinary processes of thinking, for obvious reasons of circularity.

Doctors in the past have been "religious" or vocally rationalistic in approximately equal numbers and with variations according to the fashion of the times. Religio Medici remains a classic: Maimonides was the greatest rabbinical authority of his age. Most of us who have personal religious affiliations have now sensibly learned not to obtrude them on our patients unless invited, and patients do not as a rule extend the invitation.

Now physics does not speak to religious faith: one can be a Christian, a Buddhist, a Jew or a Moslem in any of the variety of those persuasions whether "reality" consists of small hard balls or of wave-patterns. It does, however, speak—or rather, in the past it has spoken— to the picture of reality on which we project our beliefs. For example, in medieval times it was not unreasonable for believers in the concept of Heaven to place that state or location "up" or overhead. Religious ideas have to be expressed in metaphors their believers can comprehend. The problem with modern models of reality is that they are not easily visualized.

Religious faiths ("religions") are particular systems of belief and teaching: religion itself, however, is a much more general activity. The name properly applies to any attempt—dogmatic, intuitive, metaphorical, experiential or mythical—to codify the way in which our "I" relates to everything which is not-I. In this usage science itself, as well as the highly mechanistic scientism which it generated in the early part of the century, is a "religion" or general world view, which can exist in Christian, Moslem, Jewish, Hindu, Buddhist, and agnostic versions, but is still the screen on which insights taught by "religions" are projected. One could abandon some of those teachings because the metaphors in which they were expressed were antithetic to that world view and, in terms of it, simply false (Heaven could not be "up"); or one could leave the metaphors and say *credo quia impossible,* I believe *because* it is impossible, or one could look for metaphors coherent with the going climate, often to the wrath of dogmatic traditionalists.

We all know from clinical observation that "religious" patients are "good" or rewarding patients. They reward us by having inner sources of consolation and not relying on us to provide it, and by addressing death and old age with rituals and other inner and outer armaments of their own choosing. Consequently they can be left to an appropriate religious professional such as a chaplain or rabbi, and they do not force our personal confrontation with these unbiddable matters. Of course, we may have equally strong and well-systematized convictions which enable us to share their equanimity, but if not, the dying, frightened, unshriven and unshriveable patient who simply does not want to go into the dark provokes highly unpleasant countertransference reactions. Hardheaded scientism sometimes tries to cheer such patients by pointing out that they live on in their children, in humanity generally, or in their achievements, as part of a kind of moral Van Allen Belt around the rest of the world which is not terminally ill. One could not have solaced a dying dinosaur by telling him his children would one day have feathers and fly (or at least, I doubt if one could). The most helpful thing to say to our patients has been, "Where you are, death is not; and where death is, you are not." At the same time, because we are doctors, we have to see terminal illness and the last years of life, and if they make us so personally uncomfortable that we avoid them or act out in the face of them, we are bad doctors. But as the metaphors in which conventional religion expresses its brands of consolation have become more and more antique-looking, so the new understanding of what both I and That are like has the great disadvantage of being unvisualizable, and hence itself an object of metaphors, not a source from which they can be taken. Thanatological pollyanna about the wholeness of the life-cycle and death-as-experience sound uncommonly like whistlin' Dixie.

Unlike earlier medical generations, which had to deal with believers (refer to the appropriate religious authority) and unbelievers (deal with by avoidance or exhortation, if we are believers, and by reinforcing stoicism if we are not), we have to handle a wider range of attitudes. There is belief—often, in America, literalistic and fundamentalist belief in what amounts to a Biblical cargo cult—semi-belief in all its modes, stoical skepticism, badly frightened skepticism, and even the occasional seeker who has first been reassured by the doctrine of Transmigration and then scared out of his wits by the Tibetan Book of the Dead. Others, who have experimented with psychedelics, may surprise us by their conviction that "all shall be well" unsupported by a discursive theology. So far from being ready to deal with this variety, which is the human condition in microcosm, most of us are still learning to talk to the dying, and attending courses at Hospice institutions to learn that it may and should be done. After all, we share in the cultural disarray, or the excitement and uncertainty which precedes the next cultural posture. The one illicit response is to do as some of our immediate predecessors did and run from the dying patient to deal with those whom we can "cure," so as to retain the "medical reaction formation" and avoid the examination of counter-transference, which future advances in technology may hopefully postpone indefinitely.

It may, of course, be postponed or profoundly modified not so much by technology ("curing cancer", "preventing age changes": these may indeed happen, and probably will, but do not address the existential concern so much as tinker with it—people will still die on us), as by a radically new world-view which is both scientific and empathic. How far this new world view is reassuring to the nonstoical will depend on what it is seen to contain. The one major moral gain of scientific literalism/objectivism over previous philosophies was that while it was not free of denial mythologies it was not wholly programmed by the denial of personal death: in fact, by adopting a hardnosed, worst-case epiphenomenalism it was even more aggressively mortalist than the facts probably warrant. Mind was a biochemical effect dissolved with the dissolution of the objective brain, time was linear not experiential (in spite of Kant), and to believe that an individual's mental program had any ontological reality one had to be ready to believe that the Earth was flat. In this frame of mind one at least knew where one stood. The "Age of Aquarius" is likely to be a great deal more difficult—the *philosophe moyen sensuel* has got to be able to tackle quantum logic, many-worlds models, the nature of ontological "reality" in a thing-less, non-Democritean universe, and possibly parapsychology and Jungian simultaneities as well, without losing the lesson of that

Puritanical rectitude which contemplates its own mortality with acceptance, and any evidence of reservations upon it without relief. Plenty of people are already giving three cheers for transmigration, Kubler-Ross, spiritism—the theosophical lot. It is a great deal harder to treat the way forward as one of joint exploration with our patients which combines skepticism with openness.

Old age is by way of being a test of our attitudes, since medicine, which aims to postpone mortality, effectively works to *produce* old age—the period in which further postponement becomes statistically less and less feasible. From the standpoint of our own countertransference, the younger terminal patient, like the accident victim, has been unlucky, and we can avoid identification by denial (we may well be luckier). Aging, by contrast, even when we are able to retard it by intervention, will always be there, eventually to be undergone by us as well as by our patients.

Most clergymen have to deal with old people—often because in a gerontophobic society, only they and the geriatrician are available to do so. Aging is a topic with which the whole culture is uncomfortable. It is a basic threat to the American dream of controlling one's environment and living the good life, and families, where they exist, share in the experience of this threat. In the same mythology, both age and sickness are sources of religious edification. The job of religion is to deal with the unmanageables we can't control—and the role prescribed for the old is that they should acquire spiritual values as a compensation for their inability to enjoy the consumer society, die without communicating anxiety to bystanders, and leave their property to the young. By a parallel mythology, the old are "religious" in somewhat the same way that they are assumed to be asexual and disposable. As to our identifying with them and getting our own head together, we will deal with that problem when we come to it, or are terminally ill. The clergyman, who has a more caring view than that and is occupationally committed to a somewhat more comprehensive world view, has to make what educative use he can of this unpromising legacy of denial.

It is an old theory that people get "spiritual" as they age. There is no a priori reason why people should become "more spiritual" as they get older. Spirituality itself is in the nature of a fuzzy character, ranging in meaning from "more religiose" in popular usage to "more inclined to grandiloquent generalization" in pseudophilosophical usage. Genuinely "spiritual" people might well want to ditch the term in favor of a clearer definition of what their own and others' spirituality is about. What may increase with age in those susceptible to development is intolerance of triviality. This may be a fulfilling or a searing vision, according to the person on whom it falls: one of the most distressing patient-types in geriatric psychiatry is the person who has devoted life singlemindedly to the pursuit of goals which, when attained, turn out to be basically trivial. He or she is in worse shape than the man or woman depressed by failure to attain goals, because there is no recourse to any alibi.

The driving force of this late-life or terminal nontriviality of vision is the retrenchment of the sense of futurity. It occurs with aging only only on actuarial grounds: young terminal patients may experience it too. The basic component of nontriviality is the experiential conviction that all experience and activity is sacramental. Some people (William Blake, for example) appear to be born with this conviction, others achieve it, often as an uncovenanted bonus of religious or philosophical exercises undertaken for other ends. The majority of ordinary people who become "spiritual" in this sense, however, have it thrust upon them—early in life, like St. Francis, Buddha or Ramana Maharshi, by an internal confrontation with death; or later in life—like Tolstoi's *Ivan Ilyitch,* or the person approaching death through age, when denial mythologies run out.[4]

Older people are not in fact obsessed with death: such an obsession is probably commoner in children and adolescents, and sometimes in medical students of sensitivity before they become compensatorily involved in activist medicine. Awareness of mortality is a driving force of "good faith" and nontriviality, although humans only exceptionally and compulsorily use it like that: by far the most normal and practical response is denial—either by postponement or through a denial mythology. It is one of the failures of historically-oriented religions that even though probably none of their founders preached such a mythology, there has been an invincible folk-impetus to supply it: the alternative, like quantum mechanics as against Newtonian, visualizable, physics, proved too hard to explain. So while the unspiritual layman, rejoicing in the days of his youth, may do as Kingsley Amis' young man did, and deal with the thought of death by thinking quickly about sex (or some other reinforcing topic), the pious layman has been actively encouraged to deal with the thought of death by thinking about immortality—in spite of repeating every Sunday that he believes in resurrection, a very different matter.

In our culture "the old" may and do achieve a vision of the wholeness and sacral character of experience, either through or in spite of religious affiliation, but they do not get a great deal of help. Some other cultures, whose religious lives are devoted to quite a different expedient for achieving vision, offer more practical encouragement. In these, old age is a specific signal for disengagement from other preoccupations and the specific cultivation of "vision"—which classically involved dividing one's property and going to the forest, like Yajnavalkya (who took his wife with him because she too wanted the same experience).

The reason that Buddhism and Hinduism have dealt more effectively with the issue of life-cycle, death and vision than has much conventional Christianity is that, popular belief in "heaven" or "reincarnation" apart, their chief religious resource has been personal oceanic experience in which middle-order perceptions, including the homuncular, intuitivist experience of "self" and the linearity of time, are directly experienced as being conditional. Denial-mythologies do push their way into popular versions—death is only mahāsamadhi, reincarnation is just as I-centered and linear as "immortality"—but the basic relief of anxieties over cessation and not-being comes from a personal experience of the irrelevance of such anxieties to the actual form of reality. Like falling off the edge of a flat earth, they are anxieties arising from a basic misperception of the natural order, and the response to them now strikes us as scientific and empirical. It differs from science, however, in that though neuropsychology and quantum physics point to exactly the same conclusions, they are unvisualizable conclusions which do little to affect the anxieties which attend conventional, homuncular, middle-order living. Quantum physicists "know" that reality conforms rather well to oceanic intuition, but it produces few religious effects on them compared with those of direct oceanic experience. That tradition and theological set have little to do with this reordering is well shown by the results of Pahnke's experiments in inducing oceanic experience in terminally ill patients with psychedelics[2]: the experience appears to work regardless of priming, or lack of priming, from religious affiliation. Luckily, no such pharmacological assistance is needed, however: one can do the same thing more quietly.

Christianity has elected not to make great use of this kind of visionary empiricism—first, because its tradition is strongly historical, and secondly because Jesus himself, as far as any reliable records of his teachings go, did not do so. His message was of an entirely different kind, he never addressed "reality" or any other philosophical issue, his answer to the basic anxiety was to have faith in his person and follow him, and that—as Juliana of Norwich later saw in her own oceanic experience—"all will be well, and all manner of thing will be well." The wisdom of that choice in presenting a strongly ethical message to a Judaic audience in a brief ministry is borne out by the singular inefficacy of purely oceanic traditions in providing a head of ethical steam, or anything resembling Christian love, to followers who live in middle-order relationships with other people. Not many preoccupied mystics function equally well in the day-to-day mode (Blake is again a striking exception, St. Teresa another). The teaching of Jesus has been subjected to sufficient impertinent reinterpretation, but it is not devalued by suggesting that on internal evidence, his own vision was oceanic. Cornered over the dispute in Judaism for and against resurrection, he said first "I am the resurrection," then "my father's house has many rooms in it—if it wasn't so, I would have warned you" and finally "God is the God of the living, not the dead: you have got it completely wrong." The context of the last reply is that both the resurrectionists and the anti-resurrectionists, like those anxious about the edges of a flat earth, are simply asking the wrong question.

I have gone into this because I strongly suspect that most readers of this book will be Christians or Jews rather than Buddhists or Hindus, and in some cases Christians adhering to a church which has had its oceanic saints (and even its thaumaturgic yogis, like St. Joseph of Cupertino) but has assimilated them—and has been too scared of gnosticism and do-it-yourself oceanic experience to encourage it after the manner of Hinduism. It has stuck, in a practical-minded manner, to Newtonian world models (because it was talking to middle-order people it did not want to bewilder), given a strong immunizing dose of good dogma to its natural oceanics, and allowed its Hesychasts to pursue their own concerns if they found them edifying (as specialists, that is). In a world where quantum logic is of practical consequence, meditative techniques drawn from oceanic religions widespread, and a high proportion of people regard conventional models of immortality, resurrection and the like as incompatible with common sense, this simply will not serve. Christianity once stuck equally doggedly to the pre-Copernican universe for fear of making the natives restless. The natives are restless, however, and quite ready to substitute credulous versions of theosophy and spiritism for Christian or Judaic insights unless the value of oceanic experience as an educative force in perceiving the limitations of middle-order, optical, homuncular experience is taken into the club. The period of Newtonian-Huxleyan rationalism would have been unreceptive—no longer, however. We are big boys now.

As to the uniqueness of Christian or other religious insights, they have to stand or fall on their merits. Christians convinced of the value of Christian insights are not likely to stop being so convinced because of an oceanic experience: they are no more likely to become Buddhists in consequence than Buddhists are to become communicant Christians.

But given the empiricism of modern, science-oriented Man, the relative impoverishment of religious conviction based on bhaktī ("Devotion"), and the possibility of transcending the denial-mythology model of facing mortality (which, like it or not, has been as much a motive of Christian as of Eleusinian devoutness, offering a better seat in heaven to an initiated burglar than to the righteous Epaminondas), *all* purveyors of "good faith" and nontriviality in our world view need to come less anxiously to terms with oceanic vision—rather than promising their supporters "more of the same" in a hypothetical heaven extended in future-time. The model is as obsolete as the theism which worshipped a bearded old gentleman sitting on a cloud. That was primitive shorthand for primitive worshippers, and so is this. It is not only the career mystics—Juliana, St. John of Avila, Meister Eckhard—who have strayed off in this direction. Cardinal Newman's *Gerontius* looks like a Catholic journey of the soul—which it is. But it is a dream, not a prevision of postmortem experience, and dreams occur to the living: Dante's inferno contained the souls of living people, not only of the classical departed. Not only is the Kingdom of Heaven within you, real-time-wise, but so are hell, salvation and all other major spiritual experiences. If geronto-thanatologists go around canvassing Kubler-Ross shamanism as a source of reassurance in the face of mortality (although astral experiences of the kind she relies on are just as common in association with narcolepsy or after incompetent dental work under nitrous oxide as they are after near-death), the professional religionists will have only themselves to blame.

Most clergy who deal with older people are willing, unless they are monumental bigots, to play willing. They may not have a clear idea what their younger, more hip, customers are talking about, they may have a well-grounded distaste for Californian eclecticism, and most of their older flock are still comfortingly traditional. But that will change in future cohorts. Meanwhile, there is another, not directly pastoral, operation in progress, namely senior education. Droves of earnest young grannyologists—people who formerly wanted to work with children, and now, school education having run out of credit, want to "work with old people"—are moving in to live off the country. At the same time, more and more hale seniors with compulsory leisure see a return to education as a more worthwhile and less demeaning use of their time than learning to "make things out of egg boxes." At the moment, the trend is for them to view education as they always had it presented to them, à l'Américaine, as a way of getting a degree: we are seeing more and more 70 and 80-year-olds completing their Ph.D.'s. So far, nobody has realized that the educational needs of the old are different, and that meeting them may set education generally on an entirely different track. Humanities at the moment tend to mean nonuseful but fundable studies which generate degrees without the exertions required to learn science or trade.

Late age in our culture is onerous because it is "going no place." It can be lightened by renewed education—going to school, taking degrees, learning what one did not learn; these are of great help to many, but I think there is a sizable minority among the attending old who do these things rather as prisoners of war take classes in Esperanto—for the sake of something to do. At the other extreme, SAGE in California offers the whole esoteric smörgasbörd—yoga, rolfing, iridology, eurhythmics and reflexology included. This is, oddly enough, closer to what is really needed, because even fads are a way of opening congealed mental attitudes, than learning a new language one won't now get the opportunity to speak. The smörgasbörd customers for whom this bill of fare was originally designed are, however, the same as the clientele of Couch-Canyon recreational "psychiatry"—described most aptly in II Timothy 3, 6-7, as "silly women" (Paul was a male chauvinist—read 'persons') "led away with divers lusts, ever learning, and never able to come to a knowledge of the truth." For the Beverly Hills analysand, between marriages, that unamiable description is bang on target. Older people, with the opportunity to review their own track record, have passed beyond that irritable phase. What does one offer a robust, retired, hardheaded American man or woman who does not need a "shrink", has some diffuse religious convictions (often naive or fundamentalist), who is looking quite unmorbidly and without undue anxiety for an *ars moriendi* as the *terminus artis vivendi,* and doesn't want to listen to dogmatics?

Clergy (and I do not mean this offensively) are by vocation salesmen: they have convictions they want to impart. But I suggest that in dealing with American Yajnavalkyas they, like the physician, have to prepare to undertake a shared investigation. The hero figure of an empirical society is not the dogmatist or preacher but the investigator, pioneer and empiric: not believing but knowing.

The model of "going to the forest" (in which the pastoral counselor starts ex officio as guru, but may well, if he is as open and as well-grounded as most clergy today, end as co-disciple) does not involve dropping an existing framework of belief, except for those whose rigidity is such as to preclude experiential growth. Nor, of course, does it involve softheaded theosophizing in which one scrambles around other traditions looking for building materials. The highly discursive and academically intelligent could well start with a good course in modern physics. Many people already practice prayer and worship, or meditation (transcendental or otherwise). Tastes vary accordingly, and so will the mode of exploration. But the real problem is not that we live in a trivialist, godless, unphilosophical or blasé culture, but that our perceptions of the observed and observable world are basically anachronistic. Whereas Copernicus and Galileo got through to their contemporaries in relatively short order, our thinking and our perceptions are still those of 1880, and all of us, clergy and flock, are going around in intellectual frock coats and top hats. In fact, psychiatrists, who have learned to notice how their patients dress, note when the elder citizen drops his 1920's suit for a Hawaiian shirt and look for manic defense, denial—or genuine updating.

Senior education is not the same as junior education. It can involve learning new skills—such as cooking, if one can't cook, or talking Hebrew if one wants to visit Israel—but these are sideshows. The old are in their way an élite and their assignment is exploration, not the useful arts. Those who are academic enough to be philosophers can do just that (and need tapes, lectures and books to provide fuel). But SAGE, for all its fads and quacks, has the right idea. Nobody is so academically dumb that he or she cannot acquire new mental postures.

With the children whom we educate in skills, or indoctrinate with attitudes, we often wrongly assume that no experience exists. Usually this means that the experiences of childhood don't further the model citizenship we are trying to create. The old have experiences, and the first step is to bring out the experiences they have filed as educationally unprofitable or culturally unacceptable. Quite a few people of all ages, as Hardy[1] found in survey studies, have their own experiential comments on "reality" which they have kept to themselves—some of them based on experiences as compelling as those of the Oriental tradition. One hardly dares to mention "Oriental tradition" in a culture which contains enthusiasts liable to turn seniors into instant yogis on the slightest encouragement: these people's perception of the Oriental tradition is basically American-Newtonian and supermarket oriented, however. If they were psychiatrists they would aim at primal screams and deafening abreaction: if they were preachers they would want their congregation to speak with tongues. The old look on such spectacularism—which ministers to the minister, not the client—with a fairly jaundiced eye. The philosophical activities of genuine Yajnavalkyas are pragmatic, empirical, realistic, and as quiet as gardening. They have not been reprocessed by Metro-Goldwyn-Mayer in glorious technicolor, nor do they start by sitting in yogic postures. By far the best account in print of the *kind* of experimentation they involve has been given by Tarthang[3] whose suggestions would do as well for a Catholic layman or Lawrence Berkeley physicist as for a Mahayana Buddhist.* Most

*For the interested Christian priest, this book also contains the best short essay on "quantum logic" reality, by Prof. Guenther, which I have seen. A recent MIT color film on orders of magnitude, from cosmic to subatomic, reflects several of Tarthang's concerns.

clergy, keeping their eye on doctrine, would be happier, perhaps, with Meister Eckhard or the *Cloud of Unknowing,* but these are out of culture at the moment, and a less doctrinally structured language is in order. They too should examine the countertransference—are they really afraid of being forced into reeducation themselves?

One asset of the older person in achieving "spirituality" is his scepticism about professionals, which leads to a kind of openness rather like that of the modern particle physicist: he has no intellectual respectability to lose. If I were a chaplain I think I would introduce any Yajnavalkyas among my cure of souls to Tarthang Tulku, Ram Dass or Gerontius rather than the ordinary run of Christian preachers and priests. One does not want to disturb simple conviction—Jesus avoided doing so—but simple conviction is getting rarer in the climate of the times. The old have had time to assess the value they derive from the cult of their choice, to cultivate devotional experience if they are open to it, and to feel the lack of "religious experience" if they are not. All people are disconcerted by death, unless they are simply exhausted by life. Careful inquiry will usually show that there are far more natural oceanics around than have been recognized by ministers or confessors, and that a lot of doctrinally respectable devotion has oceanic origins which validate the doctrine because that is the mode of religious expression which the subject has learned. If he is a Christian, he is more likely to have the experience of Christ or Mary than of Vishnu or Mahavairocana, so the experience is assimilable: for the "irreligious" it is more open but no less compelling.

One might expect Catholics, who have a large if undervalued mystical tradition, and Chasidim, who have the Zohar, to handle this period of life better in their flock than even the most charismatic of Fundamentalists, who tend to be invincibly literal-minded and to live in a super-Newtonian universe. But since one of the gifts of oceanic experience, and a strictly nonsectarian one, is the basic revaluation of time as a part of experience, physicists and the old are probably the two groups in society most likely to make coherent use of it in reordering their world view. For the truly rationalistic, who are super-protestant in their wish to fly solo and avoid the use of figurative scaffolding, a study of quantum physics and quantum logic is itself a "religious" experience—if by religion we mean the attempt to order the relation of the experienced homuncular "I" with "That": the not-I, phenomenal reality, God, or gods, according to the meaning we attach to divinity. Only the dogmatic or the self-accusing will try to climb Mount Carmel today in the lead boots which St. John of Avila prescribed to his disciples (if he wore them himself, he got there in spite of them.) Catholics will recall that St. John's personal vision—like that of a Vaishnava devotee of Krishna—likens the religious experience to the excitement of a girl going out by night to a secret assignation.

If I, a gerontological physician of no ecclesiastical affiliation, find myself preaching a sermon here, it results not from impertinence but from experience—most recently, experience in geriatric psychiatry. I am leery of "spirituality" because I think the sacramental character of experience is general, not local, and I do not want to fuel any more comment to the effect that science is returning to "spirituality" by way of naive endorsement of old dogmatics. It isn't. But just as human mortality (and our selfish dislike of the anxiety it causes) has fuelled both religion and science, it is still the locomotive of selfknowledge in later, if not in earlier, life. The hardheaded congregations of today are not likely to be happy either with the choirs of angels or with the gibbering ghosts of the seance, and it would be a hardy Christian who adorned a modern, with-it, American church with a medieval Dance of Death. A young lady recently sent for my approval a book of entertaining sexual exercises which she described as "Tantrik"... I asked her when she last meditated in a burning-ground, an essential preliminary to the Tantrik use of sexuality in promoting oceanic experience, and got no reply. Given their head, pop-swamis and the pop-culture will trivialize Oriental insights as thoroughly as television evangelists trivialize Christian teaching. Since one of the achievements of aging is to see life as non-trivial, if we are interested in "spiritual" (non-trivial) values, we will make better use of it than that.

The epic journey of Gilgamesh was undertaken to find a cure for mortality—which, when found, was eaten by a snake. But by that time Gilgamesh had learned that he was asking the wrong question, that the preservation of "I"-ness in a mummified form by any sort of sorcery was not the real issue. Oceanic insights are immensely reassuring, but not in this simplistic way. To experience the reassurance one must have the experience—religious or sexual, scientific or devotional: the means are not especially important, nor need the result be spectacular, psychedelic or visionary. Scientists are now likely to make use of these experiences for their own (basically "spiritual") ends. The career "spiritualists" might be well advised to do the same. Even if they do not communicate these ideas to older people in search of reassurance and form in life, they will be in a better position to be of help in the resolution of the basic problem such people face.

References
1. Hardy, A.: The Biology of God, 1975. London: Cape.
2. Pahnke, W.N.: The psychedelic mystical experience in human encounter with death. Harvard Theol. Rev. 62:1, 1969.
3. Tarthang Tulku Rinpoche: Time, Space and Knowledge, Emeryville, Cal., Dharma Publ., 1977.
4. Yalom, I.D.: Existential factors in group psychotherapy. Strecker Mem. Lecture, Strecker Monogr. 11, Pennsylvania Hosp., 1974.

The Rough Beast

"Turning and turning in a widening gyre,
The falcon cannot hear the falconer.
Things fall apart, the centre cannot hold
Mere anarchy is loos'd upon the world
The blood-dimmed tide is loosed and everywhere
The ceremony of innocence is drowned:
The best lack all conviction while the worst
Are full of passionate intensity.
Surely some revelation is at hand,
Surely the second coming is at hand."

—W.B. Yeats

Bob Dylan has put it more concisely—"the times they are a-changin'." Yeats' intentions in those words were in fact right-wing and mystical, but it happens they chime remarkably well with the anxieties which we now feel about the changing sensibility, the changing style which we feel to be affecting our culture, and which most of us find difficult at this stage to analyze. I want in this chapter to attempt to examine some of the forms which this change in sensibility might take, or rather some of the considerations to which it is a response. That this is a desirable project must become obvious, I think, if we consider the nature of the last great stepwise change of this kind which we call The Romantic Movement. These large changes in our sensibility are mixed blessings. The last such change on the present scale which occurred in the last thirty years of the 18th century gave us, and I pick them at random, Blake, Napoleon, Beethoven, the guillotine, republicanism, the United States, nationalism, the democratic facade, modern industrialism, the large orchestra, Robespierre and Romantic painting. Few of these would have been accurately foreseeable in 1780 and very few of them would have been accurately assessable in 1800 even though some of them were by then physically present. The holding of seminars to unburden one's anxieties about the future was not an 18th century habit and I have failed to find in the literature any very marked discussion of the future in the years after 1770 (if one excepts the predictions of revolutionaries such as Tom Paine, or mystics such as Blake who, although they foresaw that change was coming, saw its outlines as little accurately as did Yeats in his poem). The 18th century types actually passing

211

through the Romantic climacteric realized that sensibility was changing and life was feeling different, but I believe they couldn't have written a balanced account of exactly what the changes were. Yet, within 30 years, a whole new style of human experience taking off from the shoulders of the old had introduced all of the things I just listed and a great many others.

Now I don't wish here to deprive future thesis writers in any university of material, any who may attempt to work out the interrelations between all these assorted phenomena. Relationships there certainly are between them, and they certainly make a whole, even when the phenomena are directly antipathetic in direction. The point is that here was an experience and a reaction totally different from what had gone before, and if we are on the lip of a change as radical, it would be profitable, I think, to apply ourselves to anticipate its form. There's no problem identifying a change of this kind retrospectively. It involves a complete shift in the style of a culture, whether that style is expressed in music, in science or in politics. All of these things change together and it is difficult or impossible to identify the chicken or the egg. One cannot, for example, easily confuse 18th century with Romantic poetry or painting. Obviously, there are artists like Salvator Rosa, who have been born out of their time. Erwin Panovsky has lovingly documented the ways in which the medieval treatment of classical subjects differs from the Renaissance treatment. There has been a lot of argument whether the Renaissance was a real phenomenon or whether it is something which we have invented retrospectively. All I can say is, however much one argues about detail, there is, as it were, a definite bump. It is like crossing the San Andreas Fault in an airplane. The discontinuity is there for all to see, and not only was the Renaissance view different ideologically from the medieval, but the world, viewed through new concepts of perspective in art, for example, actually came out looking different. It had come to look different exactly as the world can be made to look different to kittens who are reared in horizontally and vertically striped environments.

The change in sensibilities which we are now living through is probably at least as radical, and could be as multiple in its effects as was the Romantic Revolution. Because it is a change in sensibilities, it affects feelings and these are expressed first and explained later. As before, changes in the times are pushing whole generations into seeing the world and the world's preconceptions as radically altered. Unlike the late 18th century, however, we probably now have greater practice in our natural history, and therefore we have a much better chance of a discursive understanding of what is happening. If we can understand what is happening at the discursive level we might be able to make the consequences of the change selective. We might, in other words, be able to organize more Blakes and fewer Robespierres. It's perfectly easy and possible to make up a list of what I would term the concerns either of the pre-Romantic 1770's or of today's revolutionaries in variety. Such matters as ecology, participation, many aspects of social justice, the exploration of inner space, and so forth. I doubt if this helps us very much. The reason that we are in very great need of exposition is precisely that a revolution of this kind starts as a change in feeling. It is much easier to live it than to expound on it.

Behind it lies a great variety of experiences which are basically novel—to take a simple visual example, flight. Most of us have had a birdseye view of a city: we have seen the clouds from both sides now. With film, most of us can intuitively see a non-visual topic in terms of successive frames or of continuous motion: at the experiential level, unlike our forefathers in 1914, we as civilians have been virtually present, through television, at the Vietnam War. Although some of these experiences are difficult concepts, they feed so rapidly into our media and into our way of life that vast numbers of people can apprehend them even if they can't discourse on them or get them partially wrong—as the public of 1790 apprehended the new concepts of civil liberty even if they had not read Paine and Rousseau. Both for the academic and for the underground overtaken by this vast input of change, it is easier to recognize than to verbalize accurately and to give an indication of what it signifies other than by simply shouting. For that reason the totality of the change has few exponents as lucid as those of past revolutions, who have usually been speaking at a much later stage in the process. Also, it is given to few people living through such a revolution to see the whole of the pattern. I would suspect that Beethoven's analysis and Robespierre's analysis of what was going on would have been as different as any radical's and any conservative's analysis of what is going on today.

Revolutions are triggered when enough people suddenly realize that the current emperors and they themselves "have no clothes on." We could identify a good many of the factors which work to bring about the present matrix of change. We see vast and mindless technical expertise, some of it humane, some of it simply self-propagating. We face largely uncontrolled dangers to the entire race which arise, as often as not, simply through failing to foresee them. Central planning is essential, but authority is as irrational and vicious as ever, and bolstered in privileged countries by witless public affluence, a sort of profitless inflation at the prosperity level. Even the pigs are no longer able to provide the bacon which past generations maintained them to provide, and in all countries we have a growing educated public which has not been consulted, is resistant to traditional manipulation, and insists on having its say. That, I think, is the real crunch and it is the basis of the root and branch opting out of American youth. Faced with it, older mentors are apt to be sympathetic, expecting the opting out to be coherent and rational and then are disappointed or angry when it isn't. I think this is important because, unlike the Romantic Revolution, this one—whatever it comes to contain—is likely to prove as effective in politics as in art or in human self-estimates and though, like the Romantic, its exponents are muddled, faddy, Utopian and easily diverted, I don't see them being readily Napoleonized. The stake is too big and the emphasis on issues such as environmental politics is a potential factor in determining an abolition of politics as total as the abolition of the Divine Right of Kings and aristocrats.

To an anarchist, figures like Castro or Ho Chi Minh or Chairman Mao look less like pillars of renewed awareness than with-it and intelligent old-style politicians carried on a tide of popular courage (which, like all revolutionaries, they used for their own purposes). But then again, the same I suppose might have been said of Robespierre and Danton. Now instead of particularizing single developments or single ideological theses which contributed to the Romantic Movement, one could take a line straight through it and say that it represented a new assessment of human personality, an emergence of something we now call self-expression, the emergence of a Promethean view of man as being in conflict with the universe and in conflict very often with himself, and the idea of this conflict as a productive force. I don't feel confidence at the idea of anybody else now being competent to conduct a full-scale predictive analysis of the changes taking place in ourselves, but I think we can take a line through those in the same way and say that, at the heart of the new change in the feeling of life, is an issue of finding ways, within our culture, of achieving a viable marriage between our hearts and our heads. It is roughly a matter of attempting to find an emotional technology as sophisticated as our present enthusiasm for manipulating matter. That includes both what we call science and what we call politics.

I don't want to discourse here on "future shock." The point is that we, like the men of 1790, are beset by an enormous number of simultaneous processes. When secular changes in society come, they affect everything, from music to decency-laws and road transport facilities. We find that we have to live the changes before we can understand them—*while* understanding them, and are forced to grasp at "relevance." Ideas of relevance differ—if you are a general, what may be relevant to you is that people have stopped obeying orders: if you are a

South American peasant, what is relevant is that you are starving and your wife has a baby a year. Students rightly dissent from what academic dons find relevant: *they* may not personally be starving, but not having had time to get hardened into what is euphemistically called realism or responsibility, they nourish the quixotic idea that other people's starvation is their business: whereas the academic is more worried that standards of scholarship are changing. Both of them are right. I don't think that any concerned readers would tune me out if I go beyond the immediate relevancies and try to begin the task I mentioned, of seeing *what* is happening in just two contexts relevant to me because I practice them, politics and human biology. There is a historical, anthropological and biological package which, though it can't embrace the whole of a radical change in awareness which also includes industrial, economic and endless other matters, can come near it. Yet a change in sensibility alone, even if understood, does not necessarily make itself politically effective. It does not guarantee Blakes as against Robespierres nor preclude disasters like the Napoleonic Wars in favor of relatively successful projects like the founding of Jefferson's United States. All of these things are in the balance, and to add to them grave physical dangers not immediately related to our purposes, but related to the way we have come to live, face us both from inadvertence and from error of judgment. We have to ask whether politics, including revolutionary politics, are competent to deal rationally with these threats, even when the nature of the Newer World and its likely guidelines are known and understood.

We have to remember first that the last cultural revolution took place not only without benefit of Marx and Freud but without benefit of Darwin. Any new change in sensibility begins with a wholly different concept of Man as the substrate for any historical biology we may undertake.

I want to imagine a page of the local telephone directory, and I want you to imagine that the names set out there are the names of your ancestors—father, grandfather, great-grandfather, and so on, if those names were known. The bottom of the first column would take you back into the Bronze Age, and the bottom of the first page into remote prehistory—about 10,000 B.C. It would take between 50 and 100 pages to account for the whole of human history, depending on our definition of humanness, but almost the entire history of city cultures would be subsumed by the names on the one page. The entire scientific and technological revolution would be covered by six to ten names—say 250 years.

How far any sense of that timescale is common property I don't know. What is significant is the proportion of human formative history during which there must have obtained the virtually unchanging and highly conservative conditions of an existence very like that of the Kalahari bushman or the Australian aborigine. That is the context in which at least the evolutionary, as against the socially-acquired, portion of our human program was written.

If, accordingly, a human biologist wishes to divide society into epochs, they will not be those of the cultural historian—such as the Bronze Age, the Middle Ages, the Renaissance or the Romantic Movement. They will be related to some of the same measurables, such as attitude and technology but in quite a different distribution.

We can fairly easily observe the growth of human physical technology in matters like fire, tools and pottery. These are the general materials of archeology, but biologically speaking they are questionable criteria of humanness: apes make tools and could conceivably have made fire. Of the two human markers, no archeological record can remain. One of these is language—discursive language expressing concepts. The other is the technology characteristic of Man, which has exercised most of his talents over 90 per cent of his probable history, the technology of the emotions. The finding of artefacts does not certainly identify a level as human. Grave goods, or evidence of circumcision, for example, or the discovery of art would so identify it.

In fact the people we now describe as primitive, in that the technology they possess at the physical level has extremely little power of modifying their environment, tend in proportion to possess emotional technologies of extreme sophistication relating the individual to other humans, to animals and to inanimate objects. A large part of primitive time and intellectual energy, which is probably no different in quantity or kind from our own, is spent in activities which belong explicitly to *this* technology and only incidentally to practical activities such as hunting, crop-growing, or manufacture—the activities we term religious or magical. This is a technology which our present culture has virtually lost. I have argued elsewhere that we have today no technology of the emotions which can compare with the volume and richness of those traditional to Man. What we do have, however, are the program cards which are responsible for the structures expressed in that technology, including those which determine that at one level or another we need it.

With the vogue for structuralism in describing human behaviors, the biologist is bound to be interested in asking how far the structures which man make reflect those built-in to the generating system, the human brain. There is obviously a feedback, or rather a resonance, between the structures we make and the structures we have in us, whenever we look at a human artefact, whether literature or society. I don't intend to pursue here the use of the analysis of archetypes to work out what is in the black box. We do in fact have the possibility of externalizing these structures into another black box, the computer with which one can hold a dialogue, as one can see one's face in a mirror, but I won't evaluate that here either. My point is that the loss of this emotional technology, complementary to our socio-neurological past and present, is important, and we are only just coming to recognize it as we lose the Victorian conviction that we are here to educate the savages with railroads.

The loss is due to, or has accompanied, the contemporary sense of reality. In order to develop the scientific or empirical method on which our whole practical technology depends, it was necessary to arrive at a cultural stance in which we did not attribute smallpox objectively to devils, or believe that woodpecker's beaks cure toothache. We are just beginning to see that those "primitive" formulations possess a meaning, but for the project of control over the physical environment, which has made our lives in some respects less nasty, brutish and short, it is not the most relevant meaning. The aborigine separates them: he does not confuse the Great Ancestral Serpent with the real snakes, nor does he look for its bones, for one belongs to daily life and the other to the Dream Time. Our prosaicism was necessary for a certain type of cultural progress, as well as a certain kind of personal integrity, but very early on it is interesting to note that our religious beliefs diverged from the psychologically effective pattern of religion by getting contaminated with historicity. Not only was Christ a real person who physically rose from the dead and was tangible when He had done so; even a deeply symbolic rite like the eating of the flesh of the God had to be literalized into physical trans-substantiation, and a whole epoch of philosophy was initiated by the attempt to find an intelligible sense in which bread could become flesh without change of outward form. From that point on religion became not so much of the Dream Time, as objectively untrue, leaving us with no valid technology of feeling to replace it.

Thus literalism was essential for the acquisition of real control over nature; magic acts not on nature but on us. The overdevelopment of this part of the human potential has left us (1) without an emotional technology worth the name but (2) still in possession of the punchcards which require it, and which erupt or obtrude at all manner of points: our fathers made machines to pull trains, and found they had created mini-deities with the attributes of augustness, sexuality and personality usually programmed into ancestor-figures. We mount the exploit of physical technology par excellence in going to the moon, and find that we are repeating in detail the leading exploit of the eskimo Angakok, right down to mating with mother vehicles in space and climbing to the sky on a ladder of arrows while habited in a magic mask—even the countdown has echoes of the preliminary drumming. If you shut the door, they come in the windows!

Parallel with this loss of emotional technology, the experience of fighting against archetypal thinking in order to get practical results (what Gaston Bachelard has called thinking against our brains) has given us a civilization which possesses just as much emotional potential as our ancestors had, but with a totally reified and pseudo-rational environment in which to express it. One has to ask oneself, is New York City the practical product of technology, the rational man-made environment, or is it the reification of all the material in our minds which the primitive deals with less concretely, and possibly (though we should need to be primitives to know this) more sensibly. Are our physical structures not unwitting counterparts of Levy-Strauss-type structures which would be better dealt with linguistically or ceremonially—and if so, what about our political or our scientific structures?

If we go back now to what I mentioned about the division of history into epochs based on big human biology (by which I mean the in-depth variety, covering everything from cell chemistry to comparative religion and primate origins) we have a choice: you are probably familiar with Julian Huxley's division of evolution into stages—random, organic-genetic, behavioral and cultural, each with a different timescale. The same seems to apply within human history. The primitive has little or no capacity to modify his environment by his own technology, but a vast technology of feeling devoted to expressing his relationships with it—he experiences intense feedback from it; a kangaroo must not be killed as if it were an object, without obeisance to the spirit of kangaroos—Ayers' Rock is not merely a striking object but generative of structured relationships, as a cathedral was to the medieval peasant. The aborigine cannot control things, but tends to relate to things and animals as if they were people.

Our civilization has virtually boundless powers of direct interference with nature, and is approaching the capacity to modify some of the last inaccessibles such as the weather, by inadvertence if not by design. It experiences virtually no feedback at all from it, experiencing things totally as things. In big cities, where one passes and ignores in a morning more human beings than an aborigine meets in a lifespan, it tends more and more to reify people. In contrast to the hypothetical primitive, we tend to treat people and animals, as well as the environment, as things.

I've oversimplified this anthropologically in terms of the noble savage in order to point the nature of the change we now face: and we can
see in so doing why it is such a major change—larger in scale than, for
example the Renaissance or the Romantic Movement. If I am right, a
change of this kind—a cultural-historical one, that is—is about to coincide with a revolution of the order of that which, for example, replaced foodgathering with agriculture. The point is that science has
paid off: objective empiricism is the greatest human intellectual discovery *for the purpose for which it was intended,* namely the testing
of objective fact and the exclusion of man-made structures—even if we
perceive the printout in terms of those structures. It has paid off in that
it now can make the structures objectively visible. Whether Freud was
right or wrong in detail, his great discovery stands—that human irrationality is not random but systematic, and consequently can be read
back and comprehended. Primatology, anthropology, linguistics, and
depth psychology all fall into line. If some of them suffer from *bad*
science, that will pass: these, rather than the kind of one-cylinder market research sociology which dissident youth rightly abhors are the
real social sciences, and they are biologically based.

To oversimplify again, the primitive apparently knew how to *feel,*
and we have learned how to *think.* We now have the problem of combining the two. This is a basically scientific task, far removed from any
revisionary mysticism, which is more likely to be Nazi than enlightened. All of the concerns which make up the new revolution tend in
this direction. Even computer science, though based in hardware, con-
tributes greatly here. The introduction of feedback from things is the
difference between mechanization and automation. We sense the need
for feedback from our environment, for treating things rather more as
if they were people, at precisely the moment when brainless exploitation on one hand and engaging nuts like Mr. Buckminster Fuller on the
other threaten us with a totally man-made environment—a disaster
which, given our programming, might well be total for Man. We have
learned to use science as a protective suit, worn for thinking purposes.
We now see pathological fantasies, proper to the war gods of the
Dream Time in days when we couldn't luckily enact them, being studied "objectively" by scenario planners, and we recognize the need to
get out of the protective suit and enjoy our skins. The nudity of the
young today is a gesture of great symbolic accuracy. At one and the
same time, our discursive capacity has just about caught up with the
structure of our minds, as the irrationalities inherent in that structure
have caught up with our supposedly practical purposes—not just in
The Bomb, but in our cities, our growth economy, our environment,

our population, our attitude to our fellows, and our capacity to tolerate a steady state of accelerating change (that isn't a contradiction) with a mental economy programmed originally for a near-zero rate of social change per lifetime. It is a wonder we are as sane as we are!

I think you will see that all of the concerns of the Great Change are subsumed here, even if I don't elaborate them—anarchism instead of authoritarianism, the spaceship economy instead of the consumer society, ecology, the lot. These are concerns, not realizations. In a chapter such as this one assumes we shall pull through, as we have always done. I think that that is probably true, and that the shift which is coming will be going up a step not falling down a hole. Unfortunately, there is the new factor of time. We do not have time to reform our institutions. Institutions depend on the lifespans of ineducable people. And this may be the point of maximum danger. We retain the politics of the last century, if not of the Bronze Age, and for reasons connected with the democratic, or more accurately the show-biz method, of selecting candidates for office; for our choice of priorities modern knowledge might as well not exist. We do not, let me reiterate, need a revolt against reason, a return to God or a revival of magic, or still less any right or left-wing Jungian populism. We need a return to reason in emotionally literate terms—"inspired by love and guided by reason" was Russell's formulation, though Russell had little sense of the unconscious and the need to unravel it. And the thing which stands most solidly in the way of that is our obsolete social organization—an organization which has learned none of the insights we are now learning, and in fact rejects them with its whole being.

We live now with the political theory formulated in the last change of style, by the Romantics. And so, though only some of them realize it, do most Marxists. They have practical insights, but they are fossil insights, which explains their defensiveness against what they call revisionism and most other people call progress.

Much of the 19th century was occupied in the debate between two theories of Man, the Utopian (which argued that he was naturally sociable and corrupted only by institutions) and the wild animal (which argued that Man is a savage civilized only by the coercion of Law—propounded by other savages, it is true, but depending on the consensus effect to make it an improvement over the free-for-all which would result in cages if there were no keepers). However much these may have helped to rationalize the worries of 19th century humans faced with the need to adapt to industrialism, social revolution, and class struggle, both theories speak in categories which, for modern biology and anthropology, are quite obsolete. It is the muddle generated by this obsoleteness which comes through in the "summary issue to which all issues of the day come" as Milton Mayer called it—that of obedience to the so-called rule of Law. Don't suggest that recategorization will magically reconcile the demands for law-and-order with those of the protestors (who point rightly to the enormities which law-and-order commonly maintain de facto). In fact it may well be that such a reconciliation would remove the polarization which conventionally sparks social change in our society, the convention of reform and revolution (this of course is Marcuse's anxiety over repressive tolerance). It certainly underlies the covert anxiety of every liberal that the rigidity of authority might waver and not prove rigid enough to maintain a serviceable head of progressive steam. The point is that the game of revolution/status quo and individualism versus authoritarianism is a social convention, widespread as it has been in history. It is not the only serviceable social convention, nor is it the only playable game. It may be difficult to the point of impracticability to persuade a culture accustomed to the rules and usages of college football that (a) cricket and (b) soccer, with a spherical ball and no handling or blocking, are playable and enjoyable—in which case the convention is predictively justified. Where biology, anthropology and the like could help is in preventing the assumption that the choice of college football is an inherent attribute of human nature rather than a cultural choice.

It might or might not be profitable, and it may not yet be wise for lack of knowledge, to start the discussion of the origins of the State from primate dominance behavior, though we could perhaps start it from human family-structure, which is, as Harvey Wheeler recently pointed out, the point at which the rules of the overt, social game are learned. Early Marxists unfortunately attempted this a century ahead of any accurate knowledge either of primates or of Freud—who himself knew nothing about primates. Enough to say that there are now ethological and psychoanalytic studies which don't come very much into the political theorist's field of vision and ought to come there. All I want to say here is that the natural history of the behavior which we see in modern societies looks to a biologist or an anthropologist very different from the way it looks to the liberal constitutionalist talking in terms which would have been quite familiar to Rousseau—just as chemistry would look odd today to someone who came out of the show before Mendeleeff. Not that the constitutionalist is practically wrong: old-style metallurgy works fine. But no chemist likes to limit himself to it, and new technologies can alter it overnight.

We run head-on into the newer insights at all of the points where the older ones pinch out. The summary issue goes back to Plato: authority might be quite a different force, and far more like the necessary and normating handrail against our worser selves, if it were rational in its expressions. If it were such a handrail, it would not be the main contemporary generator of social and military abuses. One can argue that Viet Nam or Czechoslovakia represent only the aggressive drives of individual Americans and Russians representatively embodied by Authority (though this drives a sizable hole in the handrail theory). In fact, it looks as if the moral posture of governments not only in the contemporary situation but in history at large has been way behind the private morality of all but the most disturbed of their subjects, and behind that of the individual members of those governments acting privately. Hitler or Napoleon, or the Members of the Supreme Soviet, were and are privately at least tolerable. It is arguable whether their private aggressions were caged in by the State or expressed irrationally through it. Fully paid-up psychopaths of various kinds are as unregulated in their private contacts as are members of ruling groups in their public behavior (they are by definition those whom Authority fails to normate in the interests of tolerable behavior). But historically speaking, the fact seems to be that Authority (royal, dictatorial, Marxist or democratic) consists of those possessors of psychopathic drives cunning or powerful enough to embody their less-tolerable aims into the public posture of society: or alternatively that the possession of authority reveals stores of psychopathology in those who, as private citizens, manage to control them. Both are probably true. We may be wrong in thinking, as democracies do, that those who actively volunteer for office are less undesirable or more representative than those chosen randomly or by accident of birth.

The leading practical problem is, for us, that at a time when size and rate of change in society make rational organization essential to avoid overpopulation or pollution we have (a) an educated public which, having learned to take decisions on a far wider range of matters than ever before, demands to be consulted; (b) the virtual certainty that those who *volunteer* to control, e.g., our reproductive behavior will do so almost wholly for unconscious or psychopathological reasons, and will do it (if permitted) stupidly, tyrannically and irrationally; and (c) no time whatever to play around because, by adopting as our way of life a stable state of continuous change, we have left ourselves no time, whether we are radicals or conservatives. We have therefore a society which cannot act rationally, both because of the psychopathology of government and because it has no time to do the necessary planning if it were rational.

This brings me to the leading feature of government in human societies—its duality of action. There have been three characteristics of governors in all developed human societies (1) dominance and self-interest—comprehensible enough; (2) organizational duties, more or less well-done; and (3) play therapy—the opportunity for permitted acting-out. In practice and in democracies (1) and (3) usually fuse—for most rulers now, the point of staying in office is not that it confers the more normal kind of privilege (wealth, travel, women, adulation—though it does confer these things) but that it confers (3), the right to act-out unhindered. Thus for the least-normal and least-normally-self-seeking member of an administration, (1) and (3) fuse.

In the past, play therapy at the expense of society has been tolerated. The excesses of King Henry VIII or even Joe Stalin can be justified by historians on the ground that the organizational and the normative functions of a strong King were worth paying the price of a tyranny. All morality apart, this is no longer true. Organization in a modern society is increasingly the function of planners, who ex hypothesi require goals. These will normally be rational unless the public or the government make them otherwise (the rewards of being a planner or an industrial tycoon lie, for the sane, in the satisfactions of purposive activity). In our society, and for top authority, (2) is accordingly withdrawn by delegation to experts, leaving (3), play-therapy and acting-out, as the main practically observable activity of governments. In this category our modern societies include the choice of priorities. Accordingly we spend our money on going to the Moon, providing minor Supermen with their outfits and props, or hamstringing social advance in the interests of private ideology. The mechanisms are not new, but it is only with the present rate and scale of change that irrationalities in planning have become not merely miserable and uncomfortable but potentially genocidal for Man.

In our society the practical decisions "which matter" are taken by ad hoc experts. Only the choices of priorities—between moonshots and food, for example, or between the development and exploitation of other countries which presumably don't matter—are left to the play-therapy level, of governments and of corporation boards. One might think that moneymaking was of all activities the most practical if not the most lovable. If you meditate on the difference between a salary of $40,000 and a salary of $100,000, or still more between a fortune of $1M and of $100M, you will see see that this is not so. Moneymaking at this level, like political ambition, is a psychoanalytic problem, and it is part of the neglect of unconscious motives which handicapped old style marxism that it went along with the idea of rational greed as the motive of capitalist organization. It isn't. Dominance-behavior in our society is far less rational than mere avarice. And accordingly, the second great body of priority decisions, the commercial, is also left in the field of the play-therapists.

Man has always lived with unreason, but we can't live with both unreason and rapid change. Rapid change is, in fact, a new and unique rule introduced accidentally into the game by knowledge. Most human societies, whether authoritarian or open, change little and slowly under their own momentum. It has been an adaptive function of, e.g., shamans or inspired psychotics to change them discontinuously, like the Yoruba Trickster God who exists only to introduce discontinuity into the rigidity of the squarer gods, and without whom nothing new would ever happen. This stability of norm regardless of what the norm may be is a highly general human character. Most of us are programmed for it—authority as a normating force expresses rather than causes it, and it does not depend upon authority. Rather it depends on knowing where one stands. It is bad to make a new and better boat, not because King or Priest has a vested or a pathological reason against it, but because boats are made in a particular way, as everyone knows, and it is disturbing if not impious, and leading to no good, to make one otherwise unless one is a shaman inspired by Ancestor Spirits. Most of us would like things to remain as we know them. Liberals (who are overtly committed to change) would like the situation of confrontation between Reform and Establishment to remain as it was in the 19th century—as old jailbirds prefer the old-style jail, where the guards are "right bastards" to the new-style jail where they are social workers (I heard this view forcibly expressed by fellow-prisoners on many occasions when I was in jail once).

Change in everything was adopted as a pet by 19th century *progressisme* when it became a *fait accompli* of knowledge and technology. It was hard enough to control then through the old machinery, and the new machinery of stylized authority and stylized revolution (where everyone still knew where he was) was institutionalized to cope with it. But now that the rate of change is of the order of a generation or less, and still increasing, this machinery too has crumbled: there is a real difference here between the confrontations of today and those of yesterday, or last century. Kings were often pathological enough and killed people but (1) they could not kill everyone, either through malice or through preoccupation with private pathologies which made them neglect to plan; (2) the number of their subjects who had special knowledge and purposive priorities and concerns was probably smaller—our nations consist now largely (up to 25 per cent in some cases) of potential, project-oriented experts.

One expression of this is the anthropologically evident division (in England at least) between attitudes correlating with governmental office (self-styled hard-line empiricism) and attitudes correlating with knowledge (educational and psychiatric views of society). These now constitute, for us, two nearly distinct cultures, between which communication has been minimal and is now only beginning. Thus the attitude of the average high court judge and that of the average educationalist towards, say, crime are practically those of two different tribes. Inter-tribal dialogue does occur but inter-tribal hostility is high, and there are few common assumptions—in general the attitudes of the authority-group are based on arrogant rejection of knowledge, and those of the unofficial and project-orientated upon (equally arrogant) assumption of it though occasionally, as in recent "permissive" reforms, legislators have been more modern and civilized than populists. This is perhaps a tendency we could encourage by education, although (1) there is personality-selection: one can volunteer which tribe one will join, and the judge-minded subject becomes a judge, not a psychotherapist; (2) the tribes normate newcomers by the real pressures which affect social conformity, approval-seeking and status-giving, forms of operant conditioning: so that if one is a liberal and a judge one must still play at being a judge, or be disapproved—and if one is a punitive individual who somehow becomes a psychiatrist, one must pretend that one is "non-evaluative" or be an outsider. In neither of these cases does "authority" in the arm-twisting sense do the normating—such phenomena are better models of what modifies Man than the 19th century model. Nor does inter-tribal mixture work. The chaos of the American School System reflects as much the confused liberalism of teachers as the confused conservatism of authority.

We have all been disturbed by the practical impasse of administrative and popular impotence, and administrative acting-out, in the face of the exponential threats to our environment and survival. It may be that these threats will have their good effects, and resolve the problem not by exterminating us but by substituting project-orientation (so far seen only in aggressive contexts such as war) for play-therapy in office, which is an anarchist solution. Even purposive rogues would be preferable as legislators and tycoons to fanatics, however moralistic, or to the present pseudo-rational professionals—the rogue at least cares for his skin, while the austere fanatic and the principled statesman hates everyone else as much as he hates and fears himself; one might do better with the Mafia, whose motives are at least intelligibly selfish—they would have had too much sense to waste energy constructing Dachau, or computing nuclear overkill.

Non-anarchist legal theory rejects, but decent society accepts, the idea that there is an alarm button. One should go along with society up to and even a little over the edge of one's conscience: thereafter one should press the button and stop the train. The penalty for improper use is unspecified, and the propriety of button-pressing depends on split-second timing—one may be rehabilitated posthumously or not at all, depending on the machinations of the Gadarenes and the pardonable annoyance of one's fellow commuters at the delay. Gadarenes (the 1960's called them, "pigs") have no business to manipulate Law in favor of their projects; it is a fact of life that they invariably do, and it is a convention of all legal systems that the courts should pretend that they do not. It would be feasible to constitutionalize the right of citizens to press the alarm button, by appointing a tribune, ombudsman, or Commissioner for Equity, embodying the reasonable man's sense of justice, but no State has had the decency or the hardihood to appoint an effective one (it would be unpopular in the sty, where so many decisions are taken). The U.S. has gone further this way than most in creating a Supreme Court.

This is the non-anarchist, liberal-democratic model. Many are worried to know what has gone wrong—why are people pressing the button so often, and why are increasing numbers of them wanting to get off the train? Briefly, the answer is that while the democratic train is assumed to be going purposively to its announced destination, commuter opinion, backed by sound intuition, now increasingly realizes that (a) the railroad company are crooks; (b) the driver is a psychopath, or if not, may produce equally dangerous results by simply doing nothing and squabbling over business-as-usual; (c) the train is not going their way, and is probably headed for Hiroshima or Belsen. Among young commuters this evidentially-supported view is becoming widespread if not general.

The railroad by-laws, however, remain unchanged in spite of the altered situation. Piggery in office is not new—only now it is reasonably open, and unlike the piggeries of the past it has to deal with an educated, and, even in Chile or Russia, an increasingly liberal-Zeitgeist-indoctrinated public. Pigs may be no worse than ever, but the public, as a result of the independence of mind generated by many factors from science to modern education (without which there would be no science) recognizes and will no longer tolerate them. One manifestation of "science" (a new one, historically, for Man) is the objective consideration of society and its pretences, not only by occasional philosophers, but by whole publics. Mystiques such as Divine Right and the Rule of Law have had their uses, not only in roofing durable piggeries, but also in making for cohesion: Margaret Mead once convened a committee on the Ethics of Imparting Insight—she thought it dangerously upsetting. Josh Lederburg, I believe, agrees with her. Even the most milleniarist anarchists have not yet seen what seems to me the historical crunch. In a society which, by reason of its rate of change, now requires intense and rapid purposive organization, accepted "leadership" is wholly incompetent to organize anything but self-interested play therapy, and the vocal and educated New Man to whom such organization has to be sold is rightly ungovernable and demands to be consulted. We may not have *more* pigs than in the past, but they are more dangerous, more incompetent to provide even bacon and more widely recognized for what they are—in particular, as the manipulators of the literal facade of law, where some animals are more equal than others, not as the "custodians of the rule of Law" from which we all benefit. If we do not benefit, it is no thanks to them—in their book, the rule of law is strictly for the birds.

In this setting, for liberals of the old school to talk about world government is merely irritating: it could mean only bigger and better pigs acting in collusion (as they now do unofficially) instead of in competition. One Capo di Mafia may be better than multiple local goons, as a king was better than multiple robber barons, but only marginally so—he is hardly a custodian of what the modern man wants.

Such scepticism as we see about Law is only lacking in this kind of precise statement. As with the reasonable man, this is a sphere where feelings count. If it leads to the conspiratorial as against the political view of history, this in itself is a convenient empirical convention, like the electrical fluid or the Evolutionary Demon. It may not be historically true that Parliament or Congress is a body of unprincipled bastards acting with the sole objects of expressing their personal character defects, feathering their nests or staying in office. Many are as admirable individuals as the generality. But if we assume the fiction, we shall 99 times out of 100 predict correctly how they will act. It is a corollary of this that the Rule of any Law, however lovingly designed to safeguard the individual's rights, will be abused to perpetuate porcinity whenever and wherever possible, and the time will come when it will have to be militantly resisted. Indeed the wider, the less principled and the more intuitive the resistance to Authority is, the more likely is a driving-back of the frontiers of porcinity and the extension of those of just and reasonable behavior: one deserter is worth ten conscientious objectors, and one mutineer is worth ten deserters. Of course, populism can be wrong (and pigs, loath to see their kingdom fail, have a way of putting themselves at its head, as Hitler did, whether it be exasperated or revolutionary, to found new stys with different personnel). But even populism is no more often, and usually less often destructively wrong than established authority. Wars are commoner and more lethal than lynch mobs. It is up to us to make life, for future Hitlers, dangerous and brief. There are risks we must take, or stop being human. I don't think old-style liberals who are pacific and, if they will forgive me, 19th century souls, realize the stakes or take enough of such necessary risks.

The new men of 1800 were ungovernable by Divine Right. The new men of 2000 are ungovernable by anyone, though the governments of the old-style world, finding that the old-style oracles of malarkey first and force afterwards no longer work, still do not realize quite what has hit them. Optimally these new men are inner-directed—at worst they are confused and destructive; in neither event can they be "governed" in terms of conventional play-politics. And revolution is at work in all purposive or project-orientated fields—even in international industry, at least at the executive and technological level, exactly as it is among the executive and technological levels of the USSR. These are unlikely revolutionaries, perhaps businessmen and career bureaucrats—yet insofar as their concerns are practical, they must repudiate traditional nonsenses or abandon purpose. That is revolution, the revolution towards real purpose or adhocracy.

It is also, in my submission, anarchism: if the overtones of the word hamper acceptance that is partly because past anarchists have not fully realized the implications of what they were preaching. By committing oneself to non-paternalist, non-directive solutions, rather as the modern psychiatrist commits himself to non-directive counseling, one commits oneself to extreme empiricism, to non-ideology. This, in contrast to the classical Marxists, is precisely what one is obliged to do in attempting to apply science: ideology is reduced to the barest bones—we will not tolerate authority for its own sake, or its use as play-therapy: we will not tolerate solutions which override minorities or discount human emotional needs: we will not tolerate the irrational use of property, which is a special branch of power, and we will be heard—not killed off obediently through psychopathology or inadvertence. That is barely an ideology. The essence of anarchism as it now appears relevant is in recognizing that not even the anarchist's preferences may be imposed. A nondirective approach to social planning is not, fortunately, obliged to be consistent. After Marxism, after the attempt to impose bewigged parliamentary speakers on African societies, what a relief! There may be cases where it is proper to delegate or vote and cases where it is not. There are features of existing social organization which work, or which, if they do not work, are worth keeping for improvement or for fear of worse. There are others which must go. Anarchism in this sense is the only ideology which has room for the type of change we actually observe in human history, the illogical mixture of old and new. Republicans advocated the end of the Crown. What they got in Britain was an illogical compromise in which the Crown and the Peers were kept on, with varying success, to moderate the excesses of the Commons. We may well end with a mixture of anarchism and democracy ill-pleasing for neatness but empirically justified because it has grown in that way in reponse to reasonable needs and the overriding need to make power subject to protest. That protest and personal resistance, rather than coercive revolution, is the proper modality of social change is an old anarchist discovery but a new one for urban-technological Man. Existing societies will persist insofar as they find means of making that protest effective: and medicine, as the profession of responsibility to patients, not governments, is talking anarchism as Moliere's *Bourgeois Gentilhomme* talked prose.

Old-style revolutionary anarchism has come to look irrelevant to technological societies precisely by trying to be directive, to supply them with institutions to replace existing institutions. That is not its job. It loses the look of irrelevancy to developed societies immediately it concentrates, not on "revolution" as such, but on making protest effective—a role which would be just as necessary after any foreseeable revolution as before. Ex hypothesi, a society in which all valid protest was effective would not require revolution to reform it. Our style of anarchism also subsumes a more than revolutionary tolerance. Protest is not the property of those who are right, or rather left. The hardhats have their grievances too, as Marcusian as ours, and reflecting the fact that society is disappointing them: the malicious diversion by politicians of that malaise into virulent right-wing populism is a real danger, which we can defuse by understanding.

As to institutions—democracy, the Constitution of the United States, the constitution of the USSR—the attitude of this sort of anarchism is not that it is for or against them, but that they are bound to be shams unless they are made to function in spirit, as past institutional liberals purported to intend they should function, by constant and unrelenting extrainstitutional militancy. Of the existing Constitutions, that of the United States has lasted best and performed best because it has had this sanction behind it. The Constitution of the USSR has never been applied, because it has not. The consciousness of that need is today genuinely popular even where it is confused. The role of protest in substance as against paper revolution may be, to my mind, the leading political feature of the new style.

Medieval English society was much tempered, not by the Rule of Law, but by the fact that peasants were also expert archers. That situation passed, but in a sense it is returning. The power of elephantine authority has reached a point at which it is becoming less, not more. Urban technical society is highly vulnerable to popular revolt. In Britain today, the Government still talks as if it could beat a general strike by putting in middle-class blacklegs and troops. These, certainly, could deliver the mail: in 1926 they could drive trains. Not any more. The world in which fossil socialists nationalize things and fossil Tories "drive the men to heel" on the 19th century model, while fossil and decomposing foreign secretaries conclude treaties with dictators or racists to safeguard a military or trade presence in some area, is as dead as Pharaoh, and only needs a push. But whether it is any deader than the traditional preoccupations and methods of other countries, East and West, is highly arguable. United States preoccupation with weapons (while its oil lifeline is cut and its nuclear Maginot line outflanked by infantry with rifles) and foreign affairs (while its economy and morale go to hell in a handcart) is not very different.

A short way ahead of all of us—Brezhnev and Kosygin as well as Congress and Parliament—there is a canyon which is getting closer. We have not yet built any bridges. On the other side is a rational world, so far as Man is able to inhabit one—a zero-growth environmental economy, where planning is important but includes participation, where all automobiles are built like Rolls Royces because they have to be non-expendable and are bought like real estate, where there are no bigger, faster or noisier aircraft, only optimal aircraft—updated jet equivalents of the DC 3, and where research and development are geared to judgment and thought, with emotional insights thrown in, rather than up-and-over or paranoiac technology: and where, as a safety measure in case any Hitlers or Idi Amins or Stalins get any ideas, there is a militant, articulate and non-coercible public—non-coercible because it is indispensable to the complexity of life. The choice is between falling into that particular canyon and having to crawl up the other side, in the traditional way, or preparing for the transition in as orderly and rational a manner as we are able—and at least keeping the violence to a minimum. That will be difficult simply because, all ideology apart, the pattern of life—frustration with inefficiency, crowding without sociality, high input without communication, is shortening all our tempers. That may be the answer to Marcuse—prosperity of this sort does not bring contentment, still less acquiescence.

The new protest too can be irrational and act out: yet it has the current of practicality upon its side. At least it recognizes, as conventional liberalism is only now beginning to recognize, the uniqueness of the precise predicament between the need for organization and consensus and the built-in incapacity of current governments *for* rational organization. A new politics of the Environment will not necessarily be rational (it is as good a ground for demagogy and hostility as any other) but if it is indeed practical, in terms of self-interest, then it will tend to rationality, so far as that lies within the capacity of Man. And it is on rationality educated as to human emotional natural history that human survival now depends—that, and the resistance of ordinary people, paying due consideration to the non-rational side of Man, to the irrationalities of society as we now see it.

And what is the physician's political and public obligation? Certainly not to sit there yelling for preferential treatment, resisting the extension of health care for fear it may hit his pocket. Certainly not to condone frauds on Medicare because it is a government agency and fair game. Certainly not to tolerate quackery by colleagues because they are colleagues. His duty is to the patient—not to his progeny in college or his wife's desire for a bigger car; should he find this difficult he had better follow the papal wisdom and adopt celibacy, if not chastity, to cut down on competing obligations. His task (and "he", let me remind you, stands in lieu of an epicene pronoun which we lack in English—"he or she") is uncommonly difficult. He has to recognize that health care must be organized, but not allow it to be controlled by any Byzantine play-therapy group which democracy has placed in control. He should obey laws, but circumvent or ignore mere regulations. Faced with impertinent lay interference in his prescribing, he will make the diagnoses and issue the certifications needed to secure the treatment which he considers to be in the patient's best interest—but he will do this without developing a God Almighty complex, and he will elder or expel colleagues who exhibit one. He will preserve confidence—faced with demands for illicit disclosure, his memory and records will be, like the Bellman's map, a perfect and absolute blank. If asked to serve a corporation, or a body such as a prison or an army, which lays claim to allegiances which supercede direct allegiance to the patient, he will either decline as a purist, or recognizing that prisoners and soldiers need doctors, he will exercise ingenuity to preserve the correct and subvert the incorrect medical model. He will not become drunken either with wine, or with technology, or with the fantasies which he and his patients collusively promote, or with the prospect of making it to Bel Air and sitting on a million dollars while people in Watts or Harlem have no medical care.

This sounds like a prospectus for South American worker-priests, not the plump colleagues we see around us. But oddly enough, even in their Neanderthal laissez-faire, there is hope of change, for political space is curved. If you go far enough to the laissez-faire right and have even a small grain of human decency, you arrive on the anarchist Left, precisely as Marxists who suffer from a faith in government, in moving left, wind up with the Fascists on the extreme dictatorial Right. It needs only the substitution of mutual aid and direct action for laissez-faire and free competition to make anarchists even of the prosperous, if they have a conscience and are indeed members of a profession—for a profession differs from a trade in that the professional earns in order to work, and the tradesman works only to earn.

Whether the class of '80 are the leaders of a nonviolent revolution or the architects of the demise of decent medicine will depend on their choice between these roles. It will be a revolution prosecuted not with noisy demonstrations, but by the attitudes exhibited in our offices, alone with our patients, our colleagues and our ethics.